Herpes

Trusted Herpes Prevention and
Permanent Cure

*(A Complete Guide to the Medical and
Herbal Treatments)*

Pamela Smith

Published By **Jackson Denver**

Pamela Smith

Herpes: Trusted Herpes Prevention and Permanent Cure (A Complete Guide to the Medical and Herbal Treatments)

ISBN   978-1-77485-506-5

No part of this guidebook shall be reproduced in any form without permission in writing from the publisher except in the case of brief quotations embodied in critical articles or reviews.

Legal & Disclaimer

The information contained in this ebook is not designed to replace or take the place of any form of medicine or professional medical advice. The information in this ebook has been provided for educational & entertainment purposes only.

The information contained in this book has been compiled from sources deemed reliable, and it is accurate to the best of the Author's knowledge; however, the Author cannot guarantee its accuracy and validity and cannot be held liable for any errors or omissions. Changes are periodically made to this book. You must consult your doctor or get professional medical advice before using any of the suggested remedies, techniques, or information in this book.

TABLE OF CONTENTS

Introduction

People from all over the globe suffer from different kinds of herpes. Women, men, children The virus can be transmitted across them. This is further aggravated due to the lack of knowledge about the symptoms of diseases as well as cure methods and prevention strategies. Many people don't pay much focus on the condition of the lips (which is also known as "love blister") and aren't aware that this seemingly harmless "blister" when left untreated could be the source of herpes genitalis. If pregnant the herpes virus of the 2nd kind can cause serious problems that affect the development of the baby and even to the death of infants after birth. However, most people learn about it only after they've already been infected with the disease.

Genital herpes along with the virus-like effects on the gums, tongue, eyes and other parts of your body are minor problems that may develop when you're not paying attention to the herpes on your lips.

Chapter 1: What's Herpes?

Many suffer from an illness known as herpes that is caused by either HSV (Type One of Herpes Simplex Virus Herpes) or HSV-2 (Type 2 of the Herpes Simplex Virus). HSV-1 is typically connected to oral infections and HSV-2 typically is a genital infection. Recent research has revealed that the majority of HSV-1 cases are now affecting the genitals, too.

Within America, 53.9 percent of those between the ages between 14 and 49 years old have HSV-1. Just 15.7 percent suffer from HSV-2. Around 45 million people starting at 12 years old which is 1 out of 5 of those living who live in the U.S. have experienced genital HSV infection.

If you're infected by herpes it is likely that it is likely that the HSV-1 or HSV-2 virus will remain in your body for a long time. The virus is able to go dormant since it is blocked through your body's immune system. It stays in the skin's nerves. There is a chance that you will experience herpes-related outbreaks even when you have an immune system that is strong in the event that the virus begins to reproduce over and over. It is possible to treat herpes through letting it go dormant by using natural remedies. These treatments can stop and decrease the risk of herpes outbreaks that may occur in the future.

As previously mentioned, HSV-1 is transmitted via oral secretions. They are also spread through saliva, kissing or touching with the lips and the genitals or skin sores. It is also possible to transmit through sharing items that have a person who is affected by it such as dishes, towels, and toothbrushes. It is important to remember that a person suffering from herpes doesn't need to show symptoms to pass on to other people.

HSV-2 may be transmitted through sexual contact with someone with HSV-2 genital. Sexual contact may be caused by the genitals coming in contact with each other , or with the anus coming in contact with the sexual organs. In the absence of wounds or sores, the two viruses are able to be spread.

Prior to that, the majority of cases of genital herpes were caused by HSV-2. Recent research suggests that around 80percent of tertiary or college students who suffer from herpes genital sufferers also have HSV-1. This could be due to the high percentage of oral sex that is performed within this age range.

If you're pregnant and suffer from genital herpes, then it is important to discuss this with your doctor to ensure that, during the birth the baby won't be affected by the virus.

There are a variety of triggers that can cause the herpesvirus during its dormancy stage active once more. One of these is a general disease which is not serious or minor. Other triggers include fatigue and physical or emotional trauma or stress that affects the affected area , such as menstrual cycles, sexual interactions and immunosuppression due to AIDS and steroids-based medications.

Herpes is a virus that causes symptoms that depend on the type of virus the sufferer is suffering from and the part of their body the virus is affecting. Many people suffering from both types 1 and Type 2 HSV don't show symptoms in the event of an outbreak. This is known as asymptomatic illness and makes it easier for HSV to spread to others since the person suffering is unaware of the condition.

If you are suffering from oral herpes, it is possible to experience a burning, itchy and tingling or painful sensation in your lips or your mouth. It is also possible to notice cold sores around your mouth or lips. The sores could appear at first as small, open-cut ulcers, but they will become crusty afterward. The sores can last for days to weeks, before disappearing in the event that you don't treat them.

The signs of genital herpes are the sensation of burning, itching as well as a painful or tingling sensation in your buttocks inside thighs, or genital. For a couple of days, you could notice tiny blisters on your penis, vagina or anus which can rupture and cause tiny scabs that are not healing. If you are urinating and you feel an intense burning sensation when your sores are located close to the urinary tract.

Genital herpes can increase the chance of contracting HIV or AIDS. Genital sores are infected, which means that the HIV virus is able to enter your body.

Genital herpes can be found in many stages. When you contract the disease, the virus begins developing in host cells, and utilizes the cells for reproduction. There are sores and blisters within the initial few weeks following infection. this is known as an outbreak, in which the virus is present. This is the time in which herpes can be highly infectious. Your sores will be filled with viral DNA that can be transferred when touched. The virus could infect the epidermis of the skin or any other part that it comes into contact with. The initial attack usually heals within two to four weeks.

When the sores heal The herpes virus typically goes into dormant mode, where reproduction within the host cell ceases. This is where the virus becomes less transmissible. It is still important to be aware however, as the virus could be released through your skin and cause an infection. In the dormant and active stages herpes is always spreading.

If you suffer from HSV-2 and suffer an outbreak at first, you can expect to be afflicted by up to five more outbreaks over the next few years. In general, the frequency of these outbreaks decreases as time passes.

If you wish to stay clear of getting herpes-related infections and avoid transmission, try to stay away from having sexual encounters with lots of people. If you can, choose one individual as your sexual partner and be in the monogamous relationship. Your partner and you should be tested for this disease. It is also recommended to make use of condoms to lower the possibility of contracting through HSV-2.

To determine whether you're suffering from HSV type 1 or 2 it is necessary to conduct an examination in a lab on any of the sores on your body. A blood sample can be taken from you if you do not be showing any symptoms. It is used to determine if you have antibodies that are associated with your herpes virus. The blood test will determine whether you suffer from herpes and what kind you're suffering from. The test, however, will not provide a definitive answer as to which part of your body the virus affects.

If you want to be tested for herpes virus, it is recommended that you have to consult with your doctor. Although you've had the routine screening of STDs and sexually transmitted illnesses, the herpes virus might not be found unless you specifically inquire.

Keep in mind that HSV-1 is among the most widespread viruses, and there's an 80% to 60% possibility that the test will confirm that you are positive for the virus. People who are active in their sexual lives have a 10 to 20 percent chance of being negative for HSV-2.

Before getting examined for the herpesvirus There are a few things you need to consider. It is essential to understand your protection plan should you test positive in any herpesviruses. If you're negative for one of these viruses, then you need to determine if you should be aware of your potential sexual partners before kissing them, or engaging in sexual contact with them.

It can be a bit frightening and confusing to discover that you have herpes. Due to this, it is recommended that you talk with your doctor before you undergo testing to ensure you're prepared for the results of the tests.

Chapter 2: Treatment Of Herpes At Home

If you notice signs of herpes on the body that you aren't able to diagnose yourself. There are different ways to respond to the herpesvirus and most suffer from laryngosis, rashes, or sores. Since a variety of ailments can cause rashes, it is essential to be examined by a doctor to identify the exact condition you're suffering from.

After you have been tested and found to be positive for HSV-1, or 2 you may perform home treatments as part of the treatment program. The first step is to follow the basic treatment for wounds. It is uncomfortable as your blisters appear to be open and create sores or lesions. While these sores were not created by an infection, they could be infected by bacteria and become more painful for you as you fight this herpes virus. To stop this from occurring, your sores must always be free of dirt. Avoid scratching them, if you can, in order to avoid the inflammation from spreading to other skin areas. Maintain a healthy and balanced life at home to ensure that the immune system of your body is robust enough to fight infection. It is important to rest regularly and eat food that is healthy and regularly exercise.

Sores or blisters need to be treated so that they be able to dry quickly. This can be done by applying cold or cool compresses on the sores for 20 minutes. Repeat this process several times a day in order to get rid of your scabs as quickly as possible and reduce the risk of contracting a secondary bacterial infection. After your sores have become dry, you should remove your compresses since If you continue to use them your skin around the area affected by herpes is likely to dry out, leading to additional itching. Be careful when dealing with weeping blisters as their fluid is contaminated with virus that could cause chickenpox in those who have not experienced it before. If you touch the blisters or sores cleanse your hands immediately.

In addition to discomfort, herpes can trigger extreme itching. To ease this condition, apply calamine lotion to the area affected. If you've got blisters on your skin dry them off by using preparations made of aluminum acetate that is available at pharmacies. Also, you can apply aloe vera gel for calming relief. Another remedy at home is mixing half a cup of apple cider vinegar and two cups of water. A cotton cloth is dipped in the mixture, and then apply it to the area affected. It will help relieve some of the pain you experience when you have herpes.

Recent research has found the possibility that using coconut oil, in its pure form is able to help treat viral infections like herpes. Coconut oil is a source of lauric and capric acids , and studies have revealed that the oils have antiviral properties. They also fight lipid-coated virus such as HIV as well as herpes.

After consuming coconut oil the body's metabolism breaks down lauric acid into monolaurin , which is a different chemical. It eliminates viruses from each HSV-1 as well as HSV-2. When you drink 3.4 fluid 100ml of coconut oil your body produces one monolaurin, a gram. According to studies that ranges from between 3 and 9 grams monolaurin will give you a powerful antiviral effect , but it will depend on your body's chemistry and size. It is recommended to consume 10-33 ounces the oil each day for this effect. It can cause you to become sick, and negative side effects can be experienced. A better option is to consume coconut oil as a supplement that is rich in lauricidin. It is the monolaurin derived in coconut oil.

Monolaurin is a remedy for the herpes virus however it is not a cure for herpes. The symptoms are affected with this substance, specifically those who are prone to outbreaks. There are many people who have taken lauricidin for a long time and noticed lesser outbreaks. Some have even have stopped experiencing them for a lengthy period. It has the same effect of herpes medications like Valtrex. Coconut oil supplemented with is ideal for people who are not looking to use prescription drugs for herpes. Before you begin taking coconut oil, it is recommended that it is recommended to seek the advice and consent from your physician.

Recurrences usually occur following the first herpes infection. It is reported by the CDCP (also known as Centers for Disease Control & Prevention reports that four patients suffer repeated outbreaks each year. Herpes outbreaks are typically provoked by stressors, such as insomnia, stress and sun exposure as well as eating unhealthy food. It is crucial to reduce stressors in order your immune system can perform well and protect against any future herpes outbreaks.

The chapters to follow will concentrate on natural remedies for herpes, without prescription medications or drugs.

Chapter 3: Foods To Avoid And Consume

Herpes

If you suffer from herpes, following the right diet will aid in the treatment of herpes-related symptoms as well as outbreaks that are linked to this illness. Foods that are rich in the amino acid lysine, and low in arginine can help in reducing the medical issue. Lysine and arginatine are both amino acids.

When you eat food items which are rich in lysine, your herpes virus will be slowed down since the amino acid functions in a way of inhibiting. Lysine can quickly rid you of sores and extend the interval between outbreaks. The foods that contain lysine include Brewer's yeast, chicken, eggs, dairy products and legumes, organ meats, beans and seafood, as well as potatoes turkey, and vegetables.

Arginine aids the herpes virus to show up. If you're in between outbreaks the amino acid can speed up the time to the next outbreak. This can prolong the current outbreak. The most common foods containing arginine include alcohol and almonds bleached white flour chestnuts, cakes, chocolates coconut, coffee peanuts, gelatin, peanuts butter sugar, soybeans wheat germ, sunflower seeds whole wheat and white flour.

Other foods to stay clear of for those suffering from herpes include sweets, junk food and black tea as well as soda, and drinks with caffeine since they reduce your immune system. The herpes virus is able to breed, which can create a new outbreak.

There are other foods that fall to both the lysine as well as the arginine groups. They are loaded with the mineral arginine, and must be balanced with food that is rich with lysine in order for herpes outbreaks to be avoided. Consuming these food items when you are between outbreaks, and in the event that you already have an eating plan that is that is high in lysine. In the event of an outbreak then you must quit eating these foods as they could exacerbate the signs. It is possible to consume the foods again once your outbreaks have stopped. This includes bread and beans, carob cereals, chickpeas and corn Oats, peas and pancakes, pasta, rice, and others that have seeds such as tomatoes or eggplants. It is possible to eat fruit that have seeds. It is possible to eat citrus fruits but the issue is that they can cause irritation to the cold sores.

In addition to the foods you consume in addition to the food you eat, there are supplements and vitamins that can assist in the treatment of your herpes. They can help reduce symptoms and the recurrence of this condition. However, before you begin taking them you must get approval from your physician.

One of the nutrients that you must take when treating your herpes infection are Vitamin E. The vitamin assists to create healthy skin cells, and can also speed up the healing process of lesions and sores. Vitamin E helps fight infections and improves your immune system, allowing your body defend itself from the symptoms of the herpes virus. Consult your doctor if you want to use Vitamin E supplements for the treatment of herpes genitalis.

You may also utilize Vitamin C in treating your herpes as it's a powerful antioxidant. It strengthens your immune system and aids in reducing the spread of this virus. It can also help reduce the likelihood of outbreaks. Also, consult your doctor if you would like to incorporate Vitamin C in your herpes treatment regimen.

In order to reduce the duration, severity , and frequency of herpes outbreaks you can take zinc supplements. It is a metal, and is a crucial mineral to improve health. If you're not getting enough zinc, it can hinder your growth, slow the healing process from wounds and trigger diarrhea and infections. Zinc is present in lamb, beef seafood wheat germ as well as spinach, pumpkin seeds squash seeds, cashews and cocoa powder, chicken, pork as well as mushrooms and beans.

A study was conducted on people who consumed 2 milligrams of zinc sulfate a day in supplements for dietary intake. The people who took the nutrient were less likely to have a risk of developing herpes outbreaks when compared to people suffering from herpes who didn't take zinc supplements. The zinc supplemented patients had herpes outbreaks that disappeared within 24 hours, whereas those who did not supplement with it experienced the outbreaks lasted anywhere between six and 10 days.

Another study was conducted of patients suffering from herpes who put zinc oxide to the skin's surface with cold sores. Patients noticed the severity of their symptoms diminishing over a period of time. They also recovered quickly.

Medical experts agree that zinc is safe to take orally and topical use so in the dose is less than 40 milligrams daily. There are rare instances where applying zinc on the skin resulted in burning redness, itching swelling, tingling and stinging. If you notice these signs clean the zinc with mild soap and water. Don't continue making use of the solution. If you notice your symptoms worsening and persisting over three days, you must consult a physician.

If you are using the sprays of zinc for your nose, you should be aware that there have been instances where the ability for patients to smell patients was diminished. Therefore, you should be cautious when applying products containing zinc to the mucous membranes of your nose.

There are advantages to supplementing zinc in relation to your frequency and duration, or the severity of your cold sores, especially if you're zinc deficient. It is less expensive than prescription medications and produces positive results not just on herpes-related outbreaks but as well on common cold, acne macular degeneration, osteoporosis and stomach ulcers.

Absorption-wise the absorption of other minerals that zinc is competing with. These include copper, calcium and iron. It is recommended to take zinc during your meals, and keep it separate from supplements that contain minerals. If you are taking zinc along with Vitamin C the absorption will be increased. Before taking this mineral to treat your herpes infection, make sure you consult your doctor first.

The next chapter will focus on the various herbs used to combat the herpes virus.

Chapter 4: Treatment Of Herpes By Using

Herbs

Herpes treatments that are conventional include medicines like antiviral drugs. The issue with prescription drugs are that herpes viruses have been now becoming resistant to these medications. Alternative medicine and herbalists suggest trying herbal remedies with antiviral properties for treating herpes as they're more effective and more secure than conventional drugs. Before treating yourself with herbs, make sure to consult your physician for the proper instructions.

The red seaweed, Scinaia hatei, also known as scinaia, is found along the coast of India's lines is a good treatment for herpes. It is a plant that contains polysaccharides and monosaccharides. An article published in the medical journal known as Phytochemistry in August 2008 looked at the xylomannan sulfate polysaccharide water extract. The aim was to find out whether it could have anti-herpes activities. Particular kinds of polysaccharides, such as carrageenans, agarans, fucans and galactans functioned as HSV inhibitors, as reported by researchers. Xylomannan Sulfate was found in the research study to have powerful action in the fight against HSV Types 1 and 2 and virus strains that are not able to respond to antiviral drugs such as Acyclovir. Polysaccharides could impede the growth of the herpes virus , and may hinder its ability to attach to cells. In a normal dose, scinaia was not able to provide an impressive anticoagulant effect, so an increased dose may be required. It is recommended to talk to your doctor prior to taking this herb, particularly when you are taking blood thinners.

It is believed that the Indonesian evergreen tree known as eugenia caryophyllus or clove may aid in treating herpes. The flower buds are a part of the tree that has been used for cooking as well as as a medical treatment throughout the world. People of the past utilized it as a treatment for gastrointestinal problems as well as parasites, insect bites toothaches, and viral infections. The essential oil contains Eugenol which in turn has antioxidants as well as antimicrobial and sedative properties. The magazine that featured it in its "Phytotherapy Research" issue from December 2007 was a research study that examined the extracts from eugenol and clove for their ability to fight herpes. It was found that these extracts weakened the virus and slowed their replication. Within just three hours the extract of clove blocked the replication of HSV Type 1 , 2 and 3 viruses. The research supports the traditional usage of this herb for antiviral purposes. Before you use clove oil, when you are expecting a baby or with anticoagulants, it is important to talk with your doctor about the possibility of using it.

Another perennial herb that can be used to treat herpes is glycyrrhizaglabra or licorice. Its flowers are pale purple and is commonly found throughout the Mediterranean. People of the past used its dried roots to treat of liver and endocrine issues as well as skin issues, coughs and ulcers. Licorice is rich in flavonoids, polysaccharides triterpenes, volatile oil and triterpenes. It also is anti-inflammatory, antispasmodic as well as expectorant effects along with the ability to build immunity and fight viruses.

Its root is able to permanently block the herpesvirus permanently.

Medical experts recommend using a the extract or poultice of licorice if an outbreak develops due to the anti-inflammatory properties and its ability to fight viruses. You shouldn't consume licorice more than six weeks if are taking diuretics or digitalis are suffering with high blood pressure or liver issues or heart diseases, or are expecting a child.

One of the plants which can reduce the incidence and severity of genital herpes is garlic. It contains chemical compounds allicin as well as Ajoene. They have properties that strengthen the immune system, and can help to stop the spread of HSV. Garlic contains antioxidants that prevents free radicals from destroying skin cells. Before taking garlic supplements to treat signs of the genital herpes it is recommended to first obtain a permission from your doctor.

It is also possible to supplement your diet with goldenseal, an herb that can improve the symptoms of genital herpes. Goldenseal is a herb that has antibacterial and antiviral components which can reduce the impact of this virus. It is also recommended to discuss with your doctor the possibility of using goldenseal to treat the genital herpes virus.

A European plant with a lovely scent is lemon balm, and it is used for a long time by herbalists helping to treat insomnia and pain. It is rich in phenolic acids and flavonoids that are believed to fight herpes. The use of lemon balm as a topically treated treatment can help treat cold sores according to research. There is not much evidence regarding its effectiveness in the fight against cold sores that are caused by herpes genital.

If you shop at the drug and grocery shops, you'll see numerous skin care products like lotions and sunscreens with aloe vera as a constituent. There is evidence to suggest that products for the skin with aloe vera in an 0.5 percent concentration can be beneficial in the treatment of male sexually transmitted herpes.

There are numerous studies that suggest creams that contain rhubarb and sage can reduce the severity of herpes-related lesions. A double-blind study comprising the oral herpes patients of 149 was carried out. One group utilized Zovirax cream, while the other utilized sage cream. The third group utilized an ingredient in the cream, namely the combination of rhubarb with sage. The study found that the cream that contained the rhubarb and sage combination was as efficient as the prescription Zovirax cream.

Another plant that is employed internally to treat herpes is Siberian Ginseng. A clinical trial that ran for a half-year was conducted on 93 people suffering from herpes. The research suggests that using this herb could reduce the frequency, severity and duration of outbreaks of herpes. Women who are pregnant or nursing and also those with hypertension, narcolepsy, or sleep apnea are not advised to take Siberian Ginseng.

Two herbs contain compounds that fight HSV Type 1 and 2 according to research. This is the gypsy mushroom or Rozites caperata that is edible as well as Prunella vulgaris. Although the FDA hasn't given these herbs approval as treatments for herpes genitalis, it is important to be aware that they are nutritional supplements, not medicines or drugs. So, they do not need to meet the same quality standards similar to medicines that are recognized by the FDA.

If you are treating your herpes symptoms using herbal remedies, you must maintain a healthy skin. Make sure the area affected is clean and dry to speed up healing.

The next chapter will focus about alternative cures for herpes. They are all natural and do not have dangerous chemicals that many prescription medications contain.

Chapter 5: Alternate Remedies For Herpes

Herpes outbreaks can recur, and the goal is to stop them from ever returning. In addition to the natural remedies that are mentioned, which keep the herpes virus at bay for a long period of time, but not permanently There are other methods to prevent outbreaks from occurring. In this chapter, we will discuss the alternatives.

Oxygen therapy is promising for those who experience frequent Herpes outbreaks as well as painful herpes genital. The immune system could be boosted by the use of oxygen-based compound the ozone. It is also able to fight herpes virus. In order to perform this treatment less than one pint of blood is taken from you, and then infused with various amounts of oxygen and oxygen. Then, it is brought back to your veins. It is also possible to use hydrogen peroxide to combat against herpes. It is a different type the oxygen-based compound.

It is located in Europe that oxygen therapy is the most sought-after. It is also popular in the U.S., there are some states that allow doctors to administer this treatment with their patients. If you're considering using oxygen therapy, you must first know the experience of your doctor in treating herpes.

Another alternative treatment for herpes can be found in homeopathy. In this method there are a variety of common remedies, including sepia the natrum muriaticum and the toxicodendron, rhus. A practitioner of homeopathy should recommend the best treatment for you as it will be individualized to your particular situation.

If you notice blisters on the genital regions, your anus including lips and mouth, which are extremely scaly and create an aqueous fluid, look into sepia. The majority of young girls experience similar symptoms, in addition to expecting mothers, women who are menopausal and women who are experiencing menstrual cycle. In addition to these symptoms there is also feelings of sadness and weakness. When it is cold and humid conditions, their symptoms get worse.

Hepar Sulphuris calcareum can be an herbal remedy for genital herpes . These herpes causes inflammation, bleeding and extreme pain. The symptoms diminish during warmer weather.

If you experience a flare-up in your anal region, mouth, and joints that are accompanied by greasy skin, circles of eruptions, and internal sadness Try the natrum muridum. It is also a great solution if you are experiencing cravings for salt, and the symptoms become worse whenever you feel hot or uncomfortable around 10:00 in the early morning.

Also, you should look into rhus toxicodendron to help when you have blisters that encircle your mouth and genitals are itchy and burn, and also when you notice dry skin. This remedy is ideal when you are feeling agitated or when joints hurt.

Graphite may also serve as a herbal cure for herpes. You can purchase graphite pellets, which aids in the healing for various skin ailments such as herpes. Every day, consume five graphite tablets, and dissolve them in your mouth until your symptoms are gone. Graphite does not cause any side reactions that have been reported.

Arsenicum (also known as Ars alb is an arsenic that is diluted. Homeopathy experts recommend this to cure skin diseases such as herpes. It is poisonous If it is not diluted, however when it is it is diluted, arsenicum will be effective and safe. It can be purchased in tablets or pellets. If you drink coffee regularly take care with arsenicum, as any interactions can render the remedy useless. The dosage you should take will depend on the way you consume ars as well as your lifestyle.

While sulfur is used to treat acne or eczema. You can use it to treat skin irritations like herpes. It's available in small pilules or tablets. Each couple of hours, you should take several pilules in the initial dose of six. You may then have four doses daily within five days. The amount you take will be based on the sulfur type you choose to take. This remedy has not been proven to cause negative side negative effects.

If you are taking homeopathic remedies you could be exposed to a number of risks, as per homeopaths. The goal of this kind of medicine is to help balance your system by through diluted forms. If you use these for a long period however, an imbalance could develop and different symptoms might occur. In the course of two weeks homeopathy and failing to see any improvement take a visit to your homeopath and create a new treatment program.

Hydrotherapy can also be utilized to help treat herpes. Through this treatment, you apply oil to your abdomen, and then apply ice on the affected area of your genital. You may also bathe your body in warm water with salt.

The use of mind and body as a method of therapy may aid in the treatment of herpes. Herpes outbreaks usually result from stress, so it is important to find ways to alleviate stress such as meditation or guided imagery. It is also possible to join support groups for people who suffer from herpes since sharing your problems can help people feel more relaxed.

The Chinese traditionally utilized their own remedies to get rid of herpes. One of these is acupuncture, where delicate needles are inserted into specific body points to allow energy to flow smoothly. In the past, Chinese believe that when chi or energy circulates freely all over the body illness will be avoided because correct nutrients are transported across various organs and regions within the human body.

Another option to treat herpes is the capsaicin located in cayenne. It reduces the pain you experience with herpes. Find lotions or creams with this ingredient within the pharmacies and in natural health and food stores. It is also possible to use the essential oils added to the base of an oil or cream before applying it on the areas that are affected.

Another remedy for discomfort of Herpes can be found in peppermint. You can also make use of essential oils like myrrh, eucalyptus or geranium and the bergamot. Another essential oil that is popular for

Herpes treatment is tea tree. For the oils you need to dilute the chosen one with a equal amount of vegetable oil or alcohol and then apply the oil to the blisters. If you apply it on the first sign of herpes blisters, the oils could help stop an outbreak of herpes. You can also apply this treatment to treat herpes zoster, which can cause chicken pox and shingles.

There is a reason why the Echinacea plant's extract is utilized by many people to improve the capability for the body's immune system fight from infections. Some say it decreases the frequency and severity of genital herpes outbreaks. A study was conducted by researchers in the United Kingdom to compare placebo with the Echinacea effects. Five people infected with genital herpes were treated with Echinacea for a half-year and followed by placebo for another six months. Between the two time periods there was no significant distinction in the number the herpes outbreaks.

Propolis, a waxy compound produced by honeybees could aid in healing sores caused by herpes. A study was conducted with an ointment containing propolis for patients with herpes. The patients who took this ointment observed their sores heal faster contrasted to patients who were using an ointment containing either acyclovir or placebo. Patients applied the ointment onto their sores four times per day. Following 10 days of treatment, the sores of 24 out of 30 people who used propolis-based ointment fully healed in comparison to 12 of 30 who were treated with the placebo, and 14 of the 30 who applied acyclovir the ointment.

A different treatment option that has shown positive results when treating different ailments is the practice of hypnosis. A study was conducted that examined hypnotherapy in patients suffering from genital herpes . it produced positive results. The participants were from this 6-week study that showed the reduction of 50% in outbreaks of herpes and a boost in mood.

The final chapter will concentrate on the best ways to prevent herpes from returning after you've successfully cured yourself to it. This will leave you free of herpes and allow you to live a healthy and enjoyable life.

Chapter 6: Preventing Recurrences

In the final section it is crucial to understand how the herpesvirus following the initial infected. It passes through the nerve fibers of your body to reach the dorsal root the ganglia nerve. These nerves are located in these regions of your body to ensure that they won't be targeted from your body's immune system. This is due to the fact that your immune system is not able to examine this part of your nervous system.

Keep in mind that a virus's primary aim is to spread to other parasites and organisms. But since they're able to defend themselves within nerve fibers but they're not able to accomplish this purpose, so they are dormant. When your body's immune system is weak because of poor sleep, stress, or certain medicines the virus will be able to escape away from your nerves and then resurfaces on your skin. Once the virus has entered the skin your immune system is alert to it and begins attacking it. The attack causes lesions or sores. So, we can safely conclusively conclude that the virus does not cause lesions, but they are a reaction of your immune system defense against the virus.

It is crucial to safeguard the immune system against weakening to be able to avoid outbreaks of herpes. The immune system requires so many energy levels to function correctly. If you don't get enough rest and adequate nutrition your immune system is likely to be weaker. Stressing yourself mentally can cause it to wear out. Stress can cause imbalances in the body's mechanisms and chemicals, and in the beginning it attacks the energy-hungry and gentle systems.

To protect your immune system You must eat organic foods that are not processed like fruits and vegetables. You should rest each day, if you can. Also, you should relax by engaging in activities like meditation or deep breathing exercises, as well as massage. The proven methods in this book will assist you to maintain an immune system that is healthy to ensure that outbreaks of herpes be less frequent, but not completely eliminated.

If you don't treat your herpesinfection, this could make you feel uncomfortable often. Apart from these painful manifestations, you might be prone to complications. It is possible to developing HIV or meningitis, as well as encephalitis that are all serious diseases. Women who are pregnant and with herpes could suffer the misfortune of having a brain tumor or miscarriage or even her child could pass away after delivering her child to others.

To prevent the negative effects of herpes untreated You must avoid becoming infected at all. You and your partner must commit to a monogamous relationship , and you should avoid having sex with more than one partner. If you must engage in sexual sex with other people it is crucial to wear condoms made of latex. When you, or your companion displays symptoms of herpes, it's however safe and fair to engage in sexual sex at these periods.

In the end, herpes outbreaks can be prevented in the event that the immune system of your in good health through proper nutrition regularly exercising and living an uninvolved lifestyle.

Chapter 7: Herbal Remedies For Herpes

1. Tea Tree Oil for Herpes

The standard disinfectant, antibacterial, and antiviral and to fight parasites tree oil derived from the plant indigenous to Australia has established itself as a possible treatment for herpes and various bruises. If the application of tea tree oil is done every time there's any sign of an outbreak it is possible that you will see a flare-up to be out and about.

Here's the information:

Tea tree oil - 1-2 drops

Almond or olive oil (discretionary)1 - 2 tsp

Do this:

Cleanse your hands thoroughly using water and a mild cleanser and then completely dry.

If you're using tea tree oil for your skin, it is only for the reason of it, use an oil that is bearer such as almond oil or olive oil.

Mix the oil for transport with 1 drop from tea tree oil.

With the help of a dropper or cotton swabs, apply the oil to the area of your injury. Make sure not to apply the oil to different areas.

In the event that you're used to using the tea tree oil you can avoid mixing it with different oils and simply apply it to the area of injury.

After applying the oil after applying the oil, wash your hands a few times again.

Do this at least 2-4 times a throughout the day.

2. Aloe Vera Gel to treat Herpes

The gel extracted from the leaf of aloe vera is used for a variety of therapeutic purposes, among them skin disorders. Numerous clinical studies have proven that aloe vera gel is able to heal herpes-related sores quickly and effectively. Aloe vera is composed of various cell-based reinforcements and can be particularly beneficial in reducing the aggravation. It also contains salicylates that are common that help ease the pain. In addition, it's appropriate to use fresh aloe vera gel from the leaf, if possible, instead of the products which guarantee the use of aloe gel.

This is what you need to know:

Fresh aloe vera leaves (in the event you don't have this, buy pure aloe gel instead of products that say "contains aloe vera")

Blade

Do this:

Cleanse the leaf of aloe vera properly with water and wash your hands using a mild cleanser and water.

With the help of the blade, make an opening in the delicious, thick aloe leaf.

Make sure you use the blade only once more, slice the leaf of aloe and then take it out with its firm squeeze.

Apply this juice to your herpes-related bruises and bumps.

If you need to, apply a disinfected bandage or cotton swabs.

3. Goldenseal Herb for Herpes

Goldenseal is well-known in traditional drugs as a specialist in recuperation because of its alkaloids of hydrastine and berberine. Recent research has proven that berberine is anti-infection and has resilient fortifying and anticancer effects. Goldenseal is particularly effective for treating skin infections caused by viruses like the genital herpes virus or even shingles. It can be consumed as a tea, or applied topically using powder or tincture form.

How do I Utilize Goldenseal to treat Herpes?

The first method to use goldenseal in the treatment of herpes Tincture to pack

You can either use the tincture without diluting or weakening it with water to treat herpes sores.

To use it in a pure form, apply the goldenseal tincture to the herpes-infected area three times a every day.

Create a pack by absorption the tincture on a cloth.

It is also possible to apply the pack to the sores prior to settling down during the evening. It is possible to use bandage to help keep the pack up.

Remove the pack during the early part during the first day.

If you intend to use sensitive areas like sexual organs, reduce the tincture of goldenseal by adding 3-5 drops of it into a glass of water.

Then, you can splash the pack and apply it on the genital herpes lesions.

Second method of using goldenseal in herpes cure second option is to use dried goldenseal powder

It can also be used to treat both type 1 and Type 2 herpes.

You can take a small amount dried goldenseal plant powder.

Apply the powder gently on the herpes scabs and rub it into the wounds with a an emollient hand.

Repeat this three times a throughout the day.

Warning: If you're pregnant, don't apply goldenseal. Also, do not use this herb for more than fourteen days , one after the other. If it is used, provide the reprieve for at least time of 2 weeks prior to using goldenseal.

4. Oregon Grape Root for Herpes

Oregon grape root may, in fact, be described as a replacement for goldenseal plant. It is a strong ally of microbial plants that contain the germ-murdering ingredient Berberine. Additionally, it contains alkaloids that are indistinguishable from goldenseal. Chinese prescriptions use the herb extensively. Today, restorative botanists utilize Oregon graperoot, but the dried leaves of this plant have been widely used to treat various ailments, such as herpes.

This is what you need to know:

Oregon grape tincture- 1/2 - 1 tsp

Water - 1/4 - 1/2 cup

Dressing

Do this:

Blend Oregon wine tincture and water.

Take the dressing and absorb it into the water.

Look for this pack on the herpes sores you have.

Rehash 3-4 times each day.

5. Garlic is a great remedy for Herpes Remedy

Even Hippocrates who was the father of western medicine, used garlic to heal a range of diseases. Garlic is an unassuming plant easily found in every kitchen is among nature's best microbial defenses that kills a wide range of microorganisms as well as parasites, infections and parasites as well as herpes simplex 2 disease too.

The research shows that allicin-ajoene is a chemical in the plant that is found in garlic that is a powerful ingredient in killing diseases. While you may use garlic every day for your meals but make sure you use it in its crude form also. Here are some different ways to make use of garlic to heal herpes.

How do I Make Use of Garlic to treat Herpes?

The first method to use garlic to treat the treatment of herpes Sitz Bath

This is what you need to know:

Garlic bulb 1

Bubbling water-1 liter

Tub or shallow bowl

Do this:

Hack garlic cloves out of bulbs of garlic.

Sprinkle hot water over the garlic.

Give the water time to cool down to the temperature of room.

Transfer the water to a the bowl or tub. The volume of water should be enough to soak your genital area. If needed, use a bit more water.

Now, sit in the water for approximately 15 minutes.

Another method to use garlic to treat herpestreatment: Eat Raw Garlic

This is what you need to know:

Garlic cloves, 3-5

Nectar 1-2 tsp

Do this:

The garlic cloves should be taken and cut them into small pieces. You can even crush the garlic cloves or crush the garlic cloves to make glue.

Mix this garlic minced in glue or solder with sugar.

Take 2 teaspoons of this blend every daily.

When you have placed the mix inside your mouth keep the garlic in your mouth for until you're able then swallow it.

To prevent the spread of infection You can have 1 tsp of the basic garlic-nectar mix every day to help keep flare-ups in check. If you spot the primary signs of infection, begin drinking 2 tsp daily.

After you have eaten some garlic Follow it with Echinacea tea, which is our next solution at home for herpes.

Chapter 8: What Should I Expect From The

Book?

The purpose in this text is to increase your awareness and understanding of the herpes virus , with the aim of curing your illness and eliminating the herpesvirus out of your life completely. It will help you gain an understanding of the situation and offer with the confidence that you can to eliminate this awful virus! Although medical professionals might say that herpes is a permanent disease that is only treatable through vaccines and medications We believe that it is possible to rid yourself from this disease. By reading this book, you'll discover crucial facts your physician hasn't told you about and we'll supply you with the necessary tools to fight this disease, recover yourself and improve your life quality.

The most important thing to do when controlling and then getting rid of your herpes is to stay positive. Herpes will not be able to cause death! If you make the effort to increase your knowledge about the virus and follow certain measures to fight the disease, you might even be able to achieve freedom. Don't be sad about your self and don't become another statistic. Learn from this book to offer, take back control of your life and get rid of your herpes once and for all!

The Science Behind

What is the herpes virus?

The viral disease referred to as herpes is part of the deoxyribonucleic (DNA) viruses known as Herpesviridae. This group of viruses cause problems in both animals and human beings , with every member of the group being identified as herpes viruses. The name for this group of viruses is derived from the Greek word, herpein meaning "to move". This term was chosen because of the way herpes viruses cause persistent, latent infections. When it comes to the viral composition the herpes virus exhibits similar shapes when looked at under microscope. Herpes viruses comprise of double-stranded, large genomes that are linear in their nature and that contain up to 200 genes. The genomes are contained in an enclosed cage that is made of Icosahedral proteins that are referred to as"capsids. "capsid". The capsid is encased by a different layer of the protein referred to by the term "tegument" which contains both viral proteins as well as viral mRNA. This is all encased in an enveloping bi-layer of lipids known as"the "envelope". The scientific name that is that is assigned to the entire particulate structure is "virion". All herpes viruses exhibit nuclear replication tendency. This implies that viral DNA gets translated into the mRNA stored in the nucleus of the cell that is infected. The virus is infected when the particle (virion) comes into contact with the cell with specific receptor molecules that are located on the cell's surface. Once the envelope of the virus is attached to receptors on the cell membrane the virion becomes in the cell to where it is destroyed. This allows the viral DNA to spread to other parts of the cell. It is composed of the nucleus, where it begins to replicate the viral DNA. This is where the viral gene's transcription actually takes place.

There are two main herpes simplex virus families they are called HSV-1 as well as HSV-2. The viruses are also considered as of HHV-1 and 2 as an abbreviation meaning human herpesvirus 1 , and human herpesvirus 2. It is essential to recognize this distinction due to the fact that herpes simplex virus is able to affect animals as well as human beings. The causative agent for HHV-1 is for cold sores resulting from herpes and HHV-2 causes herpes genitalis. Both viruses are very widespread and highly transmissible. They are spread because of the virus shedding and reproducing through the affected body. Herpes can also be transmitted through exchanging bodily fluids, such as blood and saliva. There are eight distinct kinds of herpes viruses that can be found in people and can be passed on in various ways. They include the following:

1. HSV-1 (HHV-1) It is transmitted by close contact with an affected person.

2. HSV-2 (HHV-2) is transmitted through close contact or sexual interaction with an infected person

3. Varicella Zoster Virus (VSV) can be spread through contact with particles that are exhaled from an affected person

4. Epstein-Barr Virus (EBV) - spread through saliva of an infected individual

5. Cytomegalovirus (CMV) It is transmitted by sexual contact, bodily contact organ transplantation and blood transfusions

6. Herpes Lymphotropic virus - spread by contact with an affected person or via droplets of airborne particles

7. Human Herpes Virus 7 (HHV-7) Method of transmission isn't clearly identified.

8. Kaposi's Sarcoma-Associated Herpesvirus (KSHV) Also called HHV-8, is spread through bodily fluids, such as saliva, blood and semen.

Herpes virus appear in a variety of types, but it's also acknowledged for causing the disease for life.

The principal method through that the herpes virus achieves this is known as "immune escape" which means that the virus does not detect the immune system of humans, which allows it to endure for such a long time. One strategy for evading the immune system which the virus uses is to encode distinct proteins which mimic a protein that is referred by the name interleukin 10 that is present naturally inside the human body. Another way in which the herpesvirus is able to hide from detection is by the regulation downward of Major Histocompatibility Compatibility II (MHC II) in cells that are infected. It can occur in a variety of ways, but it all produces the same effect that is MHC is absent from its surface in the affected cell. If the MHC isn't able to reach the cell's surface, it isn't able to initiate a T-cell reaction. T-cells (lymphocytes) are activating cells in the immune system that help to detect and destroy pathogens. If the T-cells do not get activated, the herpesvirus is able to continue spreading at will.

The signs and symptoms

After you have learned the basics of the distinct varieties of herpes, and the ways they shield themselves from being detected by the human immune system, then you may be interested in learning more about how these infections affect your body.

It may also be surprising to learn that at the beginning of the course herpes can manifest with flu-like symptoms like a decreased appetite symptoms, fever, stiff muscles, swelling of lymph nodes and frequent feeling of malaise. Here you can learn more details about the specific symptoms and signs of HSV-1 as well as HSV-2.

HSV 1 Herpes simplex 1 also known as HSV-1 is commonly called oral herpes because it can cause cold sores and mouth blisters. The sores are usually tiny, fluid-filled blisters which can be quite painful, despite their size. Herpes cold cores usually appear on the mouth cheeks, lips as well as the throat and the chin, but they may be seen on the nose or on the fingers. Herpes of the mouth can be caused by HSV-1 or 2 although it is usually caused by HSV-1. While this is normal, studies indicate that HSV-1 has also been found in patients suffering from the genital herpes.

Before the sores begin to form the sores actually form, many patients report "prodromal symptoms" that is the first symptoms that precede the typical symptoms and signs of the disease. These symptoms could also include discomfort, itching or pain that lasts for an hour or so before the blisters begin to begin to appear. When the blisters begin to form they usually rupture within a couple of days and release a clear infectious fluid. Then they become crusty and remain the same until 24 hours. Herpes oral can be spread by contact with an affected person whether skin-to skin or through sexual contact. Infected people can spread the virus, even if there are no blisters The pores and skin will certainly shed the virus, without indications or symptoms. The virus typically enters the body via skin breakage and it's possible for someone suffering from the virus to transmit the virus to other areas of their body by simply touching a sore, and later touching another area or body part.

HSV-2 Herpes simplex 2 (also known as HSV-2 is commonly called genital herpes as it can cause sores that develop on the genitals, and it is most often spread via sexual contact. Although HSV-2 is the most frequently responsible for genital herpes it is also possible to transmit HSV-1 to the genital region by mouth-to-genital or sexual contact with someone with an infection of the oral cavity. Like HSV-1, HSV-2 can be transferred even if there are no sores, since the skin can shed at any moment and without or with symptoms.

In the initial week or two following being diagnosed, the majority of sufferers do not exhibit any symptoms. In the second week the first flare typically is accompanied by painful sores and flu-like symptoms. Blisters are typically found on the genitals , or close to the rectum. They crack open the leaky fluid. They then begin to crust over however it could take a few weeks for the sore to disappear. In some instances, repeated outbreaks may begin with minor symptoms like itching or tingling within the genital region. These are symptoms that are similar to those described previously for HSV-1.

The formation and size of herpes lesions are somewhat different between females and men. In men, lesions typically occur on the shaft of their penis whereas, for females, they usually appear in the vagina, the vulva and the cervix. Both genders may develop lesions on the anus, and they may affect the urethra too. Herpes genital in women typically is caused by vaginal discharge, which may transmit the virus through sexual contact with a non-infected person. One of the most alarming aspects regarding the virus herpes is it's extremely infectious but can be transmitted even if there are no signs. People with herpes may suffer from recurring outbreaks every couple of weeks, while others suffer from them once each year. When an outbreak does occur it may take weeks to heal the sores. be healed and the virus may be transferred after the sores have been healed.

People who have herpes believe that their lives are affected by the virus because there is no cure for the condition. Through this book, you'll find that there's some hope for you! Read on to find out about how you can get rid of herpes for great.

Diagnostics and Acceptance

If you're trying to reconcile the fact that you've contracted herpes, you need to look around and try to consider it as it is : an infection. If you are sick with a cold does not feel guilty for contracting a illness, and realizes the fact that his life isn't done because of it. Herpes is just another disease, and although it could alter your body in various ways, you can manage and treat it as you would with any other issue. It may take some time to get familiar with the lifestyle changes you'll need to make to avoid passing the disease, but the fact that you have herpes does not mean that it will alter your character as an individual. Actually, many patients diagnosed with herpes recognize that their condition has helped them become an improved person! If you have a condition that could be passed on to others and you must modify your daily routine to accept responsibility for yourself as well as your actions. You shouldn't continue to live in a state of mind without regard about others. You have to develop into more resilient and more compassionate person to endure the duration of herpes.

Lifestyle changes

Although the truth is that certain behavior could increase the risk of developing the disease, it is difficult to come up with a conclusion that it could be your fault for having herpes. Since herpes is a sex-transmitted disease (STI) it is a chances of contracting it increase depending on your number of partners with whom you share with. If you only have one sexual partner over the course of their lives are at a lower risk for contracting it however, it is still possible to be transmitted via contacts that are not sexual. It is crucial to keep in mind that the herpesvirus can be transmitted via a number of methods. It is possible to contract oral herpes just by drinking a glass of water with someone infected with active sores or is currently experiencing the disease. In the case of oral contact, the smallest amount of saliva may be sufficient to transmit the virus. Contrary to some STIs that are transmitted through saliva, the patient doesn't need to be afflicted with open wounds to spread the disease to an uninfected person. If the person isn't aware that they are suffering from herpes or if they know but don't inform you of the danger and it is not your fault if you contract the disease even though it's not your fault. If you have contracted the herpesvirus You should consider asking yourself some tough questions about whether it could have been avoided.

In summation:

* Being with multiple sexual partners

contact with an opened or a crusted-over sore

* Sexual activities that are not protected (oral vaginal and penetrative.)

Contact with skin during the an asymptomatic shed of the virus

* Contact with a contaminated person (touching or kissing or kissing, etc.)

The bodily fluids from an infected patient (saliva blood, semen, saliva,

* vaginal discharge)

Risk Factors for Outbreaks

In your lifetime you might experience periods of Remission. At some point, the time at where your flare-ups with herpes are referred to as "outbreaks" as well as elements that could increase the risk of having an outbreak. Some of the causes that can trigger outbreaks include:

Research has shown an association between durations of stress that are constant and repeated herpes outbreaks that are mostly seen among females. Even short-term stressors such as the aforementioned acute injury, traveling on a plane or giving an uneasy presentation at work could trigger an outbreak as well as longer-term stresses like financial concerns or ups and downs in relationships, problems in the workplace, etc.

Menstruation - A research conducted by the national institute for research in dentistry and craniofacial studies found that outbreaks of oral herpes can be caused through menstrual cycles for females. The hormonal changes that happen during menstrual cycle could cause the higher chances of an outbreak since it can be an extremely stressful time for the body and the mind. There are also some studies that suggest that the use of tampons could make genital herpes outbreaks more likely, and so can wearing tight underwear and pads for sanitary use. To decrease the risk of having a herpes outbreak during all menstrual period you can try using non-chlorinated feminine products.

Training - Exercise that is intense can be a source of stress to the body, and could affect your immune system which can lead to an outbreak of herpes. Exercise may also cause excessive sweating and chafing, which can lead to the growth of herpes lesions and sores. The milder types of exercises like walking or running are not likely to trigger an outbreak.

Dietary habits could play a crucial impact on reducing or increasing your chances of having herpes-related outbreaks. Certain foods that are the likely to cause an outbreak are alcohol, coffee nuts, chocolate the dairy industry, corn soda, and foods that are not processed. Lysine is a food ingredient which can help prevent an outbreak, however foods that contain the l-arginine (like coffee and chocolate) could actually inhibit the lysine.

Sunburn/daylight - prolonged exposure to sunlight and sunburn could increase the risk of an HSV-1-related outbreak, especially when they are combined with stress and emotional. Ultraviolet rays may hinder the function of immune cells in the pores and on the skin, that could cause outbreaks of herpes. Skin inflammation can result from sunburn and can also trigger outbreaks.

When the body's dehydrated it puts pressure on your body and the herpesvirus could profit from these weaknesses and cause an outbreak. This can happen when your lips appear dry and cracked due to dehydration. The most common dehydration-related outbreaks occur during the winter months.

Chapter 9: Medical Treatments

Let's look at some of the treatment options that are both topical and recommended for herpes:

* Topical Creams - They are available on prescription, and are used via application to the affected area. They can help to reduce the inflammation however they aren't effective in the long-term.

*Acyclovir (Zovirax) This medication helps in reducing its rate of reproduction of herpesvirus to limit the spread of its replication. This medication doesn't totally kill herpes virus. However, it does assist in reducing symptoms if it is taken for a period of 5 days.

*Valacyclovir (Valtrex) This drug can help reduce intensity of the symptoms that occur during an outbreak. This medication is only suitable for patients who are over 12 years old.

IV Medications - In the most severe of cases, intravenous medicine could be administered to ease symptoms and slow down its spread.

* Famicyclovir (Famvir) * Famicyclovir (Famvir) medication is prescribed to treat the genital herpes virus, HSV-2. It is especially beneficial for those with a an immune system that is weak.

In the event that you or your physician are certain that your illness isn't being effectively managed with antiviral medication alone, they may have suggested non-prescriptive treatments to control your symptoms. Examples of non-prescriptive options include:

1. Acetaminophen, an over-the-counter pain relief drug, is one.

2. Dietary supplements such as vitamin E that is water-soluble zinc, L-lysine and probiotics can help increase the immune system and manage the illness.

What Your Doctor DIDN'T Inform You

There are a lot of things doctors don't inform you about. Perhaps because of their ignorance or misinformation but the truth isn't being told to you. A lot of antiviral medications that are designed to ease your symptoms can cause quite unpleasant adverse negative effects. In addition they create a huge gap in your wallet! If you are thinking of donating your cash to the big pharmaceutical company, think twice and think more expansive.

Last but not least, the most important thing that pharmaceutical companies and doctors aren't going to tell you is that herpes can be treated! Continue reading to learn details about what that the medical industry of today has to tell the public about their treatment for herpes. Antiviral drugs can have side effects!

Below is an overview of of the possible side negative effects that could be experienced with Herpes medication that is widely used to treat the virus:

* Side effects of Famvir - Stomach pain, cramps excessive bleeding headaches, diarrhea.

* Valacyclovir Side Effects Depression, lack of interest, appetite loss trouble concentration insomnia, irritability headaches, ear infections, joint pain or

stiffness. Sneezing nasal congestion, sore throat.

* Acyclovir Side Effects: The stomach may hurt, swelling and weakness, fatigue, thirst and loss of appetite and decreased output of urine.

Alongside the side consequences mentioned in the previous paragraphs, there are couple of serious side effects that have been documented along with antiviral pills for herpes:

1. Acyclovir has serious crystallizing effects within the renal tube, which causes the kidney to fail.

2. In patients receiving HIV/AIDS treatment or organ transplants in conjunction with antiviral treatment.

3. Psychosis is a type of behavioral disorder that includes psychosis, mania, or delirium

4. Constipation, vomiting, nausea abdominal pain, and an upset stomach.

5. Common skin issues caused by herpes medication include rash, itching, redness

and blisters. Sometimes, they may also be associated with respiratory issues.

6. Around 50% of people suffering from herpes have headaches. Some have migraine attacks on a frequent intervals.

7. Herpes medicine has been shown to cause dysmenorrhea and painful menstrual flow.

8. Mental issues include depression anxiety, brain fog, depression and hallucinations mood swings, the irritability.

9. Other Side Effects: Heart problems, weight gain and respiratory issues, or organ failure.

The world of modern medicine might have some dark sides. Pharmaceutical companies don't wish to treat the disease; they just wish to help you manage it. The more you spend the product, the more profit they'll earn.

Rememberthat herpes is a disease that can be Curable! After you've removed the lid, you might be curious to find out the facts. A lot of the information doctors receive themselves is outdated. Doctors believe that herpes isn't a cureable disease, and therefore they treat the symptoms. There's a lot of new research that suggests that an effective treatment for herpes is feasible. Although synthetic medications aren't readily available, there are natural foods and herbs we and I can use at home to treat the condition.

It is vital to know Herpes can be a sticky virus and takes a long some time to eradicate. Thus, perseverance and persistence is the most important thing to remember.

The Step One Step

You might be wondering why you hasn't anyone told you about the cure for herpes?

The answer is easy. Big Pharma isn't willing to let you be aware of it! With time new research and new treatments are developed however, each time a condition is treated, the pharmaceutical manufacturers lose money and some of their power as well! If the general public understood that every disease could be treated using natural remedies and easy lifestyle changes they would be out of their business! We are the ones running these companies. For those who believe that illnesses aren't curable it is best to go out and conduct some research yourself, and consider a different and holistic approach for yourself.

The first step is to uncover the sheath of virus

The first step to curing your herpes infection is to remove it from hiding. In order to do this you must adhere to a strict diet plan over the course of 14 days.

In the coming two weeks, you should include the following food items in your diet

Carbohydrates are a good source of energy. They do not just provide nutrients to your body with energy but also provide

by consuming fiber. However, they can also boost your immune system.

Eat a meal of whole grain whole grain carbohydrates that are not refined at least every day -

Try to consume 7 ounces of whole grain carbohydrates at lunchtime, and between

12:30 and 12:30 and.

Dairy and Dairy Products - These food items are a natural source of lysine. It is a important ingredient.

amino acid that can boost your immune system, helping to treat sores and

stop further damage from the herpesvirus. Drink 2 glasses of milk daily to

every day to take in the daily dose of lysine two after breakfast, and one during the afternoon.

the evening before going to going to bed.

Amount of Vitamin C Foods These are foods high in vitamin C can also aid in

improve your immune system by helping it recognize and fight off the herpesvirus.

Make sure you consume two servings of citrus fruit each day (like citrus fruits like oranges) and 2 portions of

Vitamin C-rich vegetables (like tomatoes, broccoli bell peppers, broccoli, and even green

peas). Serve one serving each during lunch and another during dinner.

Healthful Fats: Healthy fats as well as omega oils can help maintain your

nervous system in good health. Try to get 1,000 mg of omega 3 fatty acids

acids.

If you are able to adhere to these guidelines for 14 days, you will observe the immune system working fully.

What can you eat?

One of the easiest methods to boost your immune system is by making easy changes to your diet. The first step is to eat foods rich high in vitamin C and the amino acid lysine. Balance your diet with carbohydrates and healthy fats is essential.

Lysine is a kind of amino acid found in many natural foods, such as dairy products. Numerous studies demonstrate the advantages of lysine in improving immunity.

Lysine is not just an extremely effective booster of the immune system and works extremely quickly too. Research on patients suffering from herpes specifically have proven that the supplementation of lysine is beneficial in reducing the frequency of outbreaks as well as reducing the time between outbreaks, for oral herpes as well as the genital herpes.

Natural food sources for lysine are:

* Cheese (Swiss/Edam cheese, 4 ounces per day)

* Salted fish (Atlantic cod 3 ounces per day)

* Nuts (pumpkin seeds, 2 cups per day)

* Products made from soy (soy 1 cup daily roast, dried frozen tofu 2 cups daily Soy chips 2 cups per day)

* Spirulina algae (3.5 ounces per day)

* Fenugreek seed (2 cups per day, cooked)

If you suffer from high cholesterol or any other cardiovascular issues, you may have to be cautious regarding increasing your intake of lysine excessively. Lysine can also boost the body's capacity to take calcium into the body, so be sure to avoid excessive doses.

Vitamin C is an additional important component of the initial step. Foods high in vitamin C may help to improve the immune system overall, while increasing the likelihood of herpes outbreaks that are extremely severe. Vitamin C doesn't just enhance the immune system generally however, it can also help to boost cardiovascular health , and may even lower your risk of stroke and heart attack. Regarding the immune system, vitamin C works as an antioxidant which assists to keep bones, blood vessels and muscles strong and healthy. Within the digestion system, Vitamin C can help to boost collagen production that assists in holding the tissues in place.

Natural food sources of vitamin C include :

* Strawberries (one cup, cut daily)

* Blueberries (3 cups per day)

* Raspberries (2 cups per day)

* Cranberries (3 cups per day)

* Kiwi (1 fruit per day, about 2 inches long)

* Bell peppers (1/2 cup daily, sliced fresh, and fresh, can be added to salads)

* Broccoli (3/4 cup per day chopped, cooked)

* Citrus fruits (1 medium orange fresh, per day)

* Papaya (1/2 medium fruit fresh, per day)

* Garlic (6 ounces per day, fresh)

* Spinach (4 cups per day cooked)

* Pineapple (1 cup per day chunks, fresh)

*Cabbage (1 half cup and 1 cup daily cooked red cabbage)

*Mango (1 1 1/2 cups daily Fresh, sliced, and fresh)

* Brussels sprouts (1 cup per day, cooked)

* Cauliflower (1 and 1/2 cups daily cooked)

* Turnip greens (2 cups per day, cooked)

* Tomatoes (3 cups per day, raw, sliced)

* Winter squash (4 cups per day, cubed, cooked)

Another supplement that can aid in strengthening the immune system Propolis. Propolis is a resin that is produced by bees. Propolis is rich in flavonoids and antioxidants, which enhance the body's natural capacity to combat harmful viruses and bacteria. Numerous studies have proven that this substance can aid to decrease the spread from HSV-1 and HSV-1 or HSV-2. Actually, these studies have proven that propolis can work faster and more effectively than antiviral prescription medications. it may also assist to ease the pain associated with herpes sores.

The magical seed: Black seed (Nigella sativa) can have magical effects for the human body. In Islamic beliefs, adding the black seed into your diet is believed to be the cure for virtually all illnesses, excluding death. In support of this the evidence, there are many reports of various diseases being treated through it. Take a small amount of seeds in the morning prior to eating anything, to help your body get stronger to its highest level. Therefore, make sure to include this into your daily diet.

Oregano Oil: Oregano oil together with other chemical compounds and methods of detoxifying our bodies, has been found to eliminate the herpesvirus. Oregano specifically kills the virus when heavy metals have been eliminated from the body through powerful detoxifiers, such as cilantro and wheat grass. However the carvacrol compound, which is a powerful ingredient found in Oregano oil applied topically and orally, has been proven to penetrate the cell membrane that herpes virus could be hiding behind and kill the virus inside the cell. Because oregano oil is stingy and is powerful it is recommended to dilute 5 drops the 'Zane Hellas' pure Greek Essential Oil Of Oregano in 1 tablespoon of olive or coconut oil, and mix it thoroughly for at least a 30 seconds. Drop 2 drops on your tongue and let it sit for about 20 secs twice every day. In addition, for application on your skin, you can take 10-15ml of coconut oil, and 2 drops of oil mentioned above and mix it thoroughly. Since herpes viruses are affixed to the root ganglion apply it on the lower back as well as the mid back every day for two times. It can be used on sores that appear on the Genitals' lips as well. The quality oil may sting in initial stages, however then the pain will ease.

(Make sure you're not taking any tablets or medications recommended by your physician prior to applying this treatment. If you must take a break from the dosage over a period of about 2 hours after the application of oil from oregano)

Below is an outline of the way these nutrients aid the immune system.

Carbohydrates are a key ingredient in an essential part in the immune system's functioning

functioning. Insufficient levels of this nutrient could result in an impairment in

such system. It is found throughout whole grains oatmeal, barley sugar, flour and

corn. If you have herpes, it's best to stay clear of refined carbohydrates, such as

white rice and white sugar because it could contain large amounts of arginine.

* Fats - - These include essential fatty acids, as well as Omega 3 oils that are extremely

Health-wise. These are known as healthy fats that are essential for health.

keeping our nervous system top shape. Foods that are high in fatty acids should be avoided to keep the nervous system in good

Hydrogenated oils are a bad choice, since they contain trans-fats, which are dangerous and can be harmful to the

body. Beware of processed and high-fat foods.

A healthy immune system is essential to keep outbreaks of herpes under control. A healthy, balanced diet, and drinking plenty of fluids will aid in fighting herpes easily and effectively. Additionally, getting enough sleep as well as reducing stress levels and exercising regularly is also important.

"Stress" - You might already be aware, stress can be an important factor that triggers herpes.

The risk of developing an outbreak is something to avoid if you are trying to get rid of your herpes. It is difficult to eliminate all stress completely from your life however, there are some ways to manage stress.

There are a few simple steps you can try to do to reduce it. Begin your day with

15 minutes of meditation in silence and don't forget to take time for yourself.

Through the daytime. Things include the practice of yoga Tai Chi, and mindful exercises

They also have been proven to also reduce stress levels.

* Exercise regularly - keeping your body in shape is a crucial part of overall health

and health. Keep in mind that moderate or mild exercising is the best for health

Herpes is a herpes-related condition when it comes to herpes. If you exercise excessively, it can trigger herpes.

Stress response in your body that can trigger an inflammation.

What NOT to Eat

Alongside increasing your intake of the amino acid lysine Vitamin C and other beneficial nutrients there are certain food items to be wary of. The three most important items you should avoid are processed food, sugar proteins, processed foods and alcohol drinks. Also, pay attention to your consumption of sulfites antibiotics, and arginine.

* Arginine-Rich Foods Nuts, peanuts gelatin and refined grains and chocolate have the amino acid arginine. Arginine is an amino acid that is essential, but it also aids in the reproduction of herpesvirus. Human bodies produce the amino acid arginine by itself, so it is best to be careful about eating.

* Sugar : Sugar can reduce the body's immune system and it interferes with the body's ability to absorb vitamin C to fight illnesses. Sugar has been shown to raise stress levels. It can cause acidity and also protects the structure of the virus. If sugar is a problem to you or very difficult to break you should check out my second book "Sugar - - The New Age Stimulant: A quick

and easy guide to Resolve Sugar Addiction as well as to Recover Yourself"

* Alcohol * Alcohol Alcohol reduces the immunity. It can trigger the outbreak of herpes. Consuming alcohol can cause the gut to be damaged and can cause cancer. It's empty calories and it reduces body nutrients. A balanced diet is essential to increase immunity and fight herpes. That's another reason to stop drinking the alcohol completely.

* Antibiotics – These drugs assist in the elimination of pathogenic bacteria however, they also kill the beneficial bacterium that helps to ensure the health of the gut and intestines. The majority of the immune system's components are located within the digestive tract, which means that having a healthy digestive system can be crucial for strengthening the immune system and fighting herpes.

* Processed Foods: Processed food items are made from artificial ingredients and have a low nutritional value. Processed food items like bottled beverages packaged foods, pre-packaged food items, snacks and

meals include preservatives, sweeteners, flavors, and colors that include Sulfites.

* Protein - Avoid from protein-rich food items. This is because protein can hinder the elimination from the virus. It causes acidity within the body. In order to treat herpesinfection, your body requires to be in an alkaline condition.

Foods to Eat

On the next pages, you will find a list of what foods you can take in the beginning 14 days in the protocol, including the days that are included within Step 1. The suggestions are intended for four days. Select at least two of them and repeat them for a number of times for up until 14 days. When you have completed Step II, you will receive additional meal ideas.

Note:

* This diet regimen is to be followed strictly without a break.

Consume as many fruits as you can. Your diet should consist mostly of fruits, and in the second place vegetables. Create

smoothies, homemade juices, and so on ...,
but do not take anything in the "do not eat"
category.

breakfast (7-10 10 am):

1. Soymilk or milk (Mandatory)

2. Fruit salad

3. Coleslaw

4. Avocado on toast.

Preparation:

For ingredients for fruit salad include: 1
medium-sized taken orange 1 cup of
strawberries and 1 cup blueberries or
raspberries. 1 medium-sized frozen kiwi,
and cream if you prefer

For Coleslaw 5 ounces of coleslaw 2
tablespoons chopped onion. 2 tablespoons
olive oil 1/2 table spoon white vinegar salt,
poppy seeds, salt.

Mix everything together in one bowl.

Avocado toast 2 slices of whole-grain bread,
toasting 1 avocado cut into slices, 1
teaspoon olive oil freshly squeezed lemon

juice 1 teaspoon, salt 1/4 teaspoon of red pepperflakes.

Sprinkle the bread with avocado. Mash avocado using the fork. Sprinkle with citrus juice and oil. Sprinkle with salt, 1/2 teaspoon and some red pepper.

Lunch

1. Fruity dessert

2. Mexican salad

3. Fruity Dessert

4. Baby spinach salad

5. Bell peppers and Soy Cheese

Preparation:

For a fruity dessert For a fruity dessert: 1 cup of strawberries or 1 cup and 1/2 mango , or 1-cup of freshly-picked pineapple.

For Mexican salad 1 avocado peeled, pitted and chopped 1/2 sweet onion chopped 1 bell pepper with a green color chopped 1 large, tomatoes, chopped, 1/2 cup fresh cilantro chopped half chopped of cilantro juice as well as salt and pepper as desired.

Combine everything into an oversized bowl and gently mix until the mixture is evenly coated.

For roasting vegetables Cubed vegetables: 1 cup squashed butternut and 1 bell pepper red seeded and diced 1/2 sweet potato cut and peeled 1 Yukon potato cubed half red onion chopped into quarters, 1 tablespoon fresh chopped thyme. 1 tablespoon freshly chopped rosemary 1/8 cup olive oil Salt and pepper.

Place the bell pepper, squash and potatoes in a large bowl. Meanwhile, in smaller bowl mix rosemary, thyme, olive oil salt, and pepper. In a bowl, toss the veggies until they're coated. Place everything in a pan for roasting and bake for up to 40 minutes.

for Strawberry as well as baby spinach For salad of baby spinach and strawberries: 2 tablespoons butter 1/2 cup of pumpkin seeds, 4oz baby spinach 1 cup of strawberry and stems cut off.

The butter should be melted in a small pan at medium-low temperature. Cook the seeds of the pumpkin. Put them in a bowl of salad and, layer the strawberries, spinach leaves and seeds. Don't put dressing until you serve. For dressing, utilize lemon juice or lime plus olive oil.

Snacks (4-5 pm):

1. Roasted chickpeas

2. Soymilk or milk (Mandatory)

3. Roasted edamame

4. Grapes

5. The seeds of pumpkin or honey.

Preparation:

To make honey: two ounces honey with soy chips or without.

Milk: 1 glass.

Grapes Two cups of grapes.

For Roasted Emamame 1 cup edamame 1 tablespoon olive oil, and depending on the taste, Powder Parmesan and salt. Or paprika or salt.

Mix the edamame with the olive oil and one of the tastes you enjoy most: Parmesan/paprika/salt -and spread them on a tinfoil baking sheet. Bake within the oven, for around 20 mins until crisp.

For roasted chickpeas: 1 cup chickpeas teaspoon olive oil, garlic powder, dried basil, 1/2 teaspoon red pepper flakes.Combine the chickpeas with oil, and seasoning.

Mix all ingredients until evenly the mixture is evenly coated. Place the chickpeas onto a baking sheet lined with tinfoil and bake them for around 20 minutes, or until crisp.

Dinner (6-8 at 7:30 pm):

1. Jalapeno and mint orange

2. Tomato soup

3. Grilled tuna served with pesto made of basil or Papaya salad

4. Broccoli and salmon or salsa

Preparation:

For broccoli and salmon A salmon fillet that weighs at least 5 ounces, grilling without oil, topped with a some fresh lemon juice and some spices according to your taste. Broccoli: 1/4 cup of chopped broccoli, cooked and served to the dish as a side dish. To make Salsa For Salsa: 2 cups chopped tomatoes 1 cup diced green bell pepper 1 cup chopped onion diced, 1 cup chopped fresh cilantro, 2 spoons of lime juice as well as salt and pepper as desired.

Grilled tuna served with basil pesto: 1 steak of tuna each weighing 8 ounces, 1/4 cup olive oils, one clove of garlic 1 cup of freshly cut basil leaves. One-eighth cup of toasted pine nuts 1 cup of grated Parmesan cheese 1 table spoon lemon juice.

The tuna should be seasoned with salt and black pepper and rub both sides with olive oil. Put it on a grill for approximately 2 minutes for medium rare, or for about 3 minutes for well-cooked. Add the garlic the pine nuts, basil leaves as well as salt and pepper in the food processor. Add the remaining oil, while blending.Transfer to an ice cube and mix in the Parmesan. Serve the tuna with.

For Papaya salad 3 cloves of garlic Fresh green pepper 3 green beans cut into 1-inch pieces 1/2 large papaya that is not ripe that has been peeled and chopped into small strips 1 tablespoon lime juice 1 tablespoon pumpkin seeds.

With the aid of a food processor, cut garlic chili peppers as well as the green beans. Mix papaya and then cut into tiny pieces. Mix in lime and tomato juice. Blend until the mixture is soft and chunky. Spice it up according to your preference.

To make Tomato soup For soup made from tomatoes: 2 tomatoes peeled and diced, two cups tomato juice 6 fresh leaves of basil, 12 cup of cream the seasonings salt and pepper.

Put tomatoes and juice into an ordinary stock pot on temperature. Simmer for 25-30 minutes. Purée the mixture of tomatoes using basil leaves, and then return the puree to the stockpot. Place the pot on moderate heat, and then stir into the cream. Sprinkle with salt and pepper.

for Orange mint, jalapeno and 2 large Oranges 1/8 cup pine nuts six mint leaves fresh, finely crushed, 1 teaspoon jalapeno that is finely chopped salt as desired, some olive oil.

Heat a small saute pan on medium-high heat. Toast your pine nuts till golden brown as well as fragrant(about about 2 mins). Transfer the nuts to a cutting board to cool. Cut off the ends of the oranges and slice the skin. Then cut each one into slices. Throw away any seeds from the orange. Serve the oranges with mint pepper and nuts, on a platter. Sprinkle salt and olive oil, if you like.

These are the food items that you should eat for the initial 14 days. Select any of the dishes depending on your preference Feel free to replace certain food items that aren't available for you. However, be sure to verify their nutrient composition prior to eating them.

The Second Step

Once you've discovered the herpes virus, the second step should be to increase the immune system. This will aid in taking care of the dissolving in the absence of virus. In this stage of the treatment, you'll concentrate on the most important nutrients, supplements, and other food inclusions.This phase lasts between 11 and 13 days.

1. The Olive Leaf Extract It is a potent extract is made up of elenolic acid as well as an elenolic salt, also called calcium elenolate. It is extremely effective in fighting against the herpes virus. The dosage of this extract is typically determined by the oleuropein content. Try to take two capsules of 500 mg made of extracts from the olive tree 4 times every day during meals for adults or two capsules of 500 mg each the day to children. It is best to spread your doses over the course of breakfast dinner, lunch snack and dinner.

2. Alkaline purified water - Drinking lots of alkaline purified water is vital to detoxify and supply nutritious nutrients. Dehydration can trigger for herpes. For the best results drinking alkaline or distillate water since it has been cleansed to eliminate the majority of chemical toxins as well as others harmful elements. Try to drink at eight glasses of alkaline drinking water every day. The more the more effective! Alkalinity aids in detoxification and helps to suffocate herpes viruses. Acidic however, creates the

creation of a healthy environment for the herpes virus.

3. Supplements Boost your Immunity through taking Lysine (2000 mg daily) and Vitamin C (4000 mg daily) non-acidic supplements. One good example is "Non acidic Vitamin C Powder Sodium Ascorbate Non GMO Fine Crystals that dissolve in water for a healthy immune system as well as Cell Protection, Antioxidant and Health". It is easily available in online stores, such as Amazon.

A myth: A large dose of vitamin C will not cause health problems, it gets absorbed by urine. Make sure you are well-hydrated.

This will aid in healing sores, lessen outbreaks and maintain the health of your heart and brain. The supplements can aid in recovering from stress.

If you adhere to this method for between 11 and 13 days you will notice that your body is completely free in the battle against the herpesvirus! It's as easy as that. In the pages to follow, you will get more specific instructions on how to implement this solution.

A healthy daily routine

Making healthy adjustments to your routine, you will increase your immunity and increase your body's capacity to fight against herpes. The three essential elements that you should include in your daily routine include olive leaf extract, lots of water, and health supplements.

Drink daily herbal extracts You can think about herbal extracts such as Echinacea as well as prunella vulgaris. Echinacea is a natural remedy proven to reduce the duration and severity of cold viruses and prunella vulgaris has been proven to aid in treating herpes viruses in particular. Use the dosage as indicated on the label on the back of the bottle.

Reduce stress with calming foods The information you've received is about the necessity of reducing stress when fighting the herpesvirus. You'll be amazed to find out that certain foods help you fight stress. B vitamins have the ability to increase the activity of the nervous system and help to create an "feel great" hormone called serotonin . that helps your body and mind to be relaxed and comfortable. Food sources for B vitamins are dairy products such as whole grains, fresh green fruits, mushrooms, salmon and tuna.

Breakfast Suggestions to Second Step

The next steps will require between 11 and 15 days. Apart from taking your lysine, vitamins C, vitamin B or the capsules of olive leaf extracts The main issue for everyone following this plan is the diet. Keep in mind: Drink as much plenty of water, as much as is possible. In the area of diet it is not as if you're so much conditioned like you were in Step I, since you're now on the full supplement-mode. Enjoy whatever you wish to eat throughout the day, and avoid, of course , items listed in the "NO list" however, you should begin your day by eating breakfast. eating for between 11 and 15 days, with one of the suggestions below. You are able to try any of them, or choose three or more to do them over between 11 and 15 days.

Breakfast plan (7-10 Am):

1. Fruit Salad

2. Soup with cold parsley

3. Toast and mushrooms

4. Cesar Salad with Smoked Salmon

5. Fennel Salad

6. Cucumber Salad

Preparation:

For fruit salad For salads: 1/2 peeled medium size orange 1 cup of fresh pineapple and 1/4 chopped strawberries. 1 cup blueberries 2 Table spoons with honey.

Mix them up and serve.

Morning cold soup with parsley 1-medium leek (white and green portions only) 1 large bunch freshly flat-leaf parsley(1/4 1 pound) 2 tablespoons of olive oil 1 medium zucchini(1/2 1 pound) removed and cut in cubes of 1/2 inch, salt water.

Chop the leek into pieces and wash in a bowl cold water. Mix it. Then, lift out and dry. Leeks and parsley are cooked in oil on a moderately low heat, stirring occasionally until they soften, approximately 5 minutes. Add salt and zucchini, and cook, stirringfor for 1 minute. Add water and simmer under cover, for about 10 minutes, or until the zucchini is tender, approximately 10 minutes. Blend the mixture with the parsley leaves to make it smooth.Season by adding salt and pepper.The recipe makes several servings. Consume only one medium-sized bowl.

Toast and mushrooms Toast: 8 cups olive oil 1 garlic clove 2 table spoons of parsley fat-leaf leaves chopped 1 teaspoon thyme leaf chopped, 1/2 lemon and rind, finely grated. two large, flat mushrooms, stalks trim and 2 slices of whole-grain bread 1 teaspoon Parmesan.

Grill should be heated to high temperature. Combine garlic, oil, parsley the thyme, lemon's rind, the salt and pepper into a a bowl. Place mushrooms, with the stems facing down, on a grill tray and serve with bread. Massage the mushroom in olive oil. If you wish you, add some herbs. Grill for three minutes. Turn the mushrooms over and toast them. Brush the mushrooms once more, then on the opposite side. Sprinkle Parmesan over the the top. Grill for another 3-4 minutes, or until that the mushroom is cooked and the bread has been cooked and the Parmesan melts.

Cesar salad with Smoked salmon: 1/4 medium-sized lettuce, 2 pieces whole grain bread 1 tablespoon of light mayonnaise, juice of 1.5 lemons, 1 tablespoon mustard 1 cup yogurt milk and 3oz file-smoked salmon. Parmesan cheese, and salt to taste.

Place some olive oil in the pan, then put in the Parmesan cheese. Once the cheese is golden, reverse the cheese into the bowl, creating this shape. Combine all of the components together for the dressing. Cut the toast into cubes, then bake the oven to bake until it gets crisp. In the cheese, simply put the salad. The salmon should be placed on top.

Fennel salad: five ounces of arugula washed and dried 1 small bulb of fennel, thinly cut 2 tablespoons olive oil. Three tablespoons lemon juice as well as pepper and pecorino (not necessary).

Mix the arugula with the Fennel in a serving bowl. Include lemon juice, olive oil salt, and pepper on the top. Add pecorino cheese and serve with olive oil.

Cucumber salad 1/8 cup red onions chopped 1 tea spoon honey 1 1/2 cups of cucumbers with seeds. 1/8 cup of fine cut red peppers. Half teaspoon sesame seeds. 1/4 cup of olive oil.

Mix everything up and then enjoy!

The Final Step

In the final stage we will cleanse the body of the remnants of the virus.

The only way in which toxins mucus, parasites bacteria, viruses and mucus could go away is when it is joined with oxygen. The body cannot be cleansed unless oxygen is in the body. The purpose of detoxing is to get more oxygen! If your body is alkaline, your hemoglobin can absorb more oxygen from your lung. Alkaline is required for your body and numerous body functions, specifically on a cell level. If the body is able to absorb increased oxygen, everything performs optimally, from energy production to detoxification and the elimination of harmful bacteria and viruses. The body is greatly benefited in the event that it's acidic or more, it utilizes oxygen at a higher rate. You must understand that on a cell scale, cells require oxygen to convert sugar to ATP within mitochondria. If you don't have enough oxygen, your body won't be able to eliminate metabolic waste, won't create H_2O_2, and can't eliminate heavy metals and toxic substances.

Here's a wonderful cleanser juice that you can consume. It's not the greatest tasting but neither does herpes.

Use a handful of dandelions, cilantro, and watercress into a blender and put 500-750ml of water into it. Blend it thoroughly and consume all day long. Test the amount of greens in your own.

This oxygen- and detoxifying drink can help eliminate the contaminants from your body. will take in oxygen and help to build the healthy function system in your body. The drink doesn't need to be consumed prior to the conclusion of the two first steps, but it can be included in the first two steps.

The thing to keep in mind is that when treating herpes, you must go to the source. The more attentive you are about your diet and the more quickly you can get rid of it! Be aware that eating excessive fruit cures all diseases. Patients have healed themselves in a month, two months, and some even 2.5 months. The key is patience!

Chapter 10: Understanding The Medical

Technemes As Well As Generalities In

Genital Herpes

Healthy appetite for and active sexuality isn't only a modern idea of life, but also one of the most essential and beneficial requirements to keep your biological clock running. In the same way that sexual Education has served as the biggest source of information for our time, it has been accompanied by a plethora of new sexually transmitted illnesses and infections that are as harmful as our own enlightenment to sexuality!

The first time you are introduced to sexuality, it will be a bit immature, regardless of age however, as time goes by, it's important to know the proper precautions and other information to ensure your sexual health is in good condition. Nowadays, even with tenfold attention and care, some diseases are able to get past the protection of our protocols. One such sexually transmitted disease that's stuck in the state of "with" or "without the possibility of a cure' can be Genital Herpes.

A virus known as Herpes Simplex The virus transmits Genital Herpes or HSV II and I. Genital herpes typically announces its presence in the body via cold sores , lesions or pustules in the genital area. The virus we are aware can cause infections within our bodies, when it is in contact by. HSV is known to infiltrate the body of the body of an affected person via simple activities, as well as through sexual interaction and through the mouth. Typically, the suffering and pain caused by herpes can be severe when left untreated because of the inevitable frequent Relapses. A person with a herpes infection could experience between 5 and 6 instances each year. The affected area can vary in proportion to gender, as well as other genetic aspects.

As with many STI (Sexually transmitted Infection)s of old age, Genital Herpes has a subset of the STI that could be fatal if it is untreated. The subset of herpes that is known as Neonatal Herpes and Herpetic encephalitis. The first is a threat to newborns while the second is being studied.

Different types of Herpes

Herpes has been described by the past as a disgusting and embarrassing illness due to its severity and frequency based upon the health and sexuality of an individual. The illness causes vesicles, or blisters on the genital region in four to seven days following contact with an infected person but, for some it could go undetected!

Genital herpes is caused by Herpes Simplex virus (HSV) which is part of the herpes virus family , which causes human genital herpes. The two most common viruses cause Genital Herpes,

1. Herpes Simplex Virus-1

This virus can cause cold sores among patients suffering from herpes. The infection is infectious and is transmitted by saliva, mucus lesions, or even through casual contact. It can cause Oral herpes, and is believed to have a biological connection to Alzheimer's in addition to Genital Herpes. The theory suggests that this kind of virus affects the nerve system an individual by preventing the lipoprotein inhibitors. This virus does not cause herpes genital as HSV is a possibility to contract early in the child's life and can cause genital herpes. The virus is found in the ear during the initial stage, before it begins to multiply or shedding out from there.

2. Herpes Simplex Virus 2

The nature of contagiousness and transmission in the second class of HSV is identical to HSV 1 with the exception of the location of the affected areas. In general, when a patient is identified by HSV-2, blisters and lesions are typically located in the genital region and on the rectum, or beneath the waist. HSV II virus settles at the base of the spine and then begins to multiply or explode into the genital region to spread the virus.

Fertility, Pregnancy , and other options when living with Genital Herpes.

Genital herpes is among the conditions that aren't hereditary due to an array of biological mechanisms that are employed within our own body. Genital Herpes is not transmitted through the ovary or sperm and therefore are not a hindrance to the reproduction capacity of the body.

It isn't any problem for a woman suffering from herpes genitalis. This is due in part to the fact that both pregnancy, and labourare both an array of trillions of antibodies injected to the mother's blood to safeguard the baby inside. However, the concentration of the affected parent must be raised following the birth because infants are at an increased likelihood to contract the disease due to touching, kissing and other contact. But the danger isn't that severe, because herpes virus usually will wane and dies if not being in close contact with cells.

If you are aware that you have herpes isn't yet known, visit to a physician and speak with them, to obtain all the explanations and details you require about the same. Genital herpes is an awe-inspiring experience as well as an untruthful term to all those who are paranoid! There are many counsellors who offer a seasoned level of help, in case your troubles and issues are in no way resolvable at the moment. to help you find authentic treatment, therapies and methods for the assurance of being free of herpes.

Signs and symptoms of Genital Herpes

Genital herpes typically causes painful symptoms such as blisters, pustules, and lesions when it first appears however, in some instances, they can be symptoms that are not present. Because genital herpes has become an extremely common STI for the majority of adults nowadays, the most important thing to remember is to check your body with an accredited physician to establish evidence that can be used immediately to receive all prompt medical treatment. After acquiring herpes simplex virus from an affected person, the symptoms begin to appear in two weeks or. Here are some of the signs of genital herpes.

1. Tingling

2. Itching

3. Lesions or blisters in the Genital Area

4. Lesions or blisters in the inner thighs or elsewhere beneath the waist

5. Mouth sores that are cold such as anus, rectum or on the genitalia

6. Unusual vaginal discharge or stinky discharge

7. Red-spots and painful ulcers

8. Painful Urination

9. Joint pains and fever

10. Stress and depression

The cervix vagina, clitoris, as well as the labia are often the first to be affected by the development of red, painful spots.

For males the penis's shaft, anus, rectumand foreskin and tip of penis are affected by blisters or lesions that are filled with water or pus.

For some experiencing the first herpes outbreak, it could be so painful that they not have another outbreak throughout their life! In other cases, herpes outbreaks occur every 5 to 6 years. In the course of the outbreak, blisters will reappear in infected regions and fade in approximately 20 days.

The recurrences are a sign of Genital Herpes

In accordance with the frequency of herpes outbreaks that occur in an entire year, a physician prescribes medication to the patient. If a person has a herpes infections less than six times per year, they are provided with an episodic treatment. If a patient has more than six herpes outbreaks each year, the doctor recommends a treatment for suppression. Recurrence is one of the most important aspects of the genital herpes. This recurring Herpes genitalis can be known as recurrences. They tend to be less severe than the initial outbreak. The frequency of recurrences will vary based on the individuals. Herpes genital recurrences can be described as follows

1. The genital region or on the legs prior to the beginning of the outbreak

2. The appearance of blisters in clusters in the genital region

3. Cold Sores

4. Lesions

5. Pimple-like red spots

6. Ulcer development and healing via the creation of a crusts over the ulcer

Recurrences tend to be less severe than the first outbreak. as with each flare, the body generates greater and greater amounts of antibodies in blood to combat HSV. Therefore after an extended period, frequency of recurrences decreases and even non-existent. The catalysis factor for outbreaks could be as high as tonnes and range in severity from issues of anxiety, depression, loneliness drinking excessively, and exposure to sunlight procedures in the genital area, or triggers for immune weakening. The Herpes virus is not able to disappear from the body once infected. It will never leave the body. The virus is able to remain dormant inside the body until an outbreak occurs. This is why it is essential to be checked by a doctor when you suspect the presence of genital herpes. Furthermore the immune deficiency of patients with genital herpes may be a sign to have an examination for HIV too.

The causes and the frequency of Genital Herpes

To understand the main factors that lead to being infected by Herpes Simplex virus, one must recognize that we all have herpes virus based on our history that includes shingles or chicken pox (herpes Zoster). The causes of battling Genital herpes is through skin-to-skin contact with a person who is infected via oral, anal and vaginal contacts. The skin areas that are sensitive to take in moisture, absorb the herpes virus from areas of the genital area, resulting in the genital herpes. The initial episode can last for three weeks and is characterized by an itching sensation and tingling sensation that will eventually turn into groups of lesions or blisters. These warning signs are medically known as prodromes. They then transform into ulcers , and eventually crusts that are healed in a period of 2 to 3 weeks. There are some stages that be present without prior ones and result in just cut or damaged skin. Joint pain and fever are the most common symptoms of herpes the recurrence.

Modern Treatment Methods to Treat Herpes

Since Herpes Simplex virus is one of the viruses that will does not go away once it has entered and is among the STIs that are not curable in a perfect way. However, there are some natural cures and precautions adhered to with a strictness, to keep the number of cases to a minimum. The virus stays dormant within the root ganglia spine of our bodies to develop into a full-blown herpes genital infection at some point. The virus can undergo two transformations when it is infected by the herpesvirus cells. These are:

1. When the Herpes virus is able to penetrate cell walls, it will begin to rupture and explode within the body, spreading the HSV into the bloodstream and thus increase the risk of transmission that causes Genital Herpes.

2. The other way that HSV will behave to undergo multiplication. The rapid multiplication process can weaken the immune system of the body in the presence of the virus.

When it is discovered that there is HSV within a person the first action to be taken by a physician is to stop the disease from spreading further by providing antibiotics to boost the body's immune system. The antibiotics are given in an average dose of 2000 mg for 7 to 7 days. The typical antibiotics prescribed for those identified with the genital herpes

1. Acyclovir

2. Famciclovir (Famvir)

3. Valaciclovir (Valtrex)

A different method of treatment is based on the amount of outbreaks that a person is diagnosed with Herpes must fight. Because herpes remains among the diseases that is incurable the treatment options are to keep the outbreaks at minimal levels and decrease the effectiveness of the condition every time an outbreak occurs. The consumption of the medication for Genital Herpes, confirms the reduced rate of spread of the disease to a lesser extent or none at all.

1. Episodic Treatment

This treatment is available to patients who do not have more than six Herpes episodes per year. It is designed to control the numbness or sensation of tingling before the full-blown beginning or prior to herpes Recurrences. This method of treatment is called Episodic Treatment.

2. Supressive Treatment

This treatment method is recommended to patients suffering from more than six cases from Genital Herpes per year. It is also recommended to patients suffering from severe physical and mental distress caused by Genital Herpes. The treatment is focused on reducing the severe outbreak pattern by using higher doses of medication to reduce the risk of the spread of infection. The aim of treatment is to prevent the possibility of a new outbreak of the disease. The patient is given some of Genital Herpes antiviral medicines for an entire year, taking the usual dosage of two pills daily. It also lowers the chance of transmitting an STI to your companion. The treatment usually lasts throughout the year, as each infection is less severe than the preceding one. If the problem becomes serious the patient will need to undergo a further medical exam to determine if there are any other signs of impairment to the immune system.

The most recent Methods of Treatment

The most recent treatment for genital herpes concentrates on stopping the spread of the STI instead of treating it. One of the initial steps to determine the best treatment for a particular patient who is infected of Genital Herpes is to conduct thorough examinations or checks of the body and immune system. The first test to confirm the severity of infection are through three primary methods. They are:

1. The PCR Test of Blood

The most precise and accurate Genital Herpes test to recognise the extent of infection studying the DNA for Herpes Simplex Virus present in the body is known as PCR test of blood. This test can detect an outbreak of Genital Herpes after the healing process and crust development.

2. Cell Culture

The test is carried out by removing a portion of pus or blisters that are present in the area of infection then analysing it using taking it to be culturing. Professionals with experience then examine the slide using microscopes for evidence of HSV.

3. Antibody Tests

They are the tests that can be used in the future to determine if you have the presence of genital herpes. The test considers how much antibodies that are produced following contact with the virus. The solution is analyzed for luminescence following the mixing of the fluorescent dye with HSV antibodies, which result in an ethereal glow along the edges of the slide solution, after being examined under the microscope.

The two tests that are first performed can result in negative or False positive results. The tests do not provide the exact time of the infection, however they do reveal the additional health issues, the extent and nature of the infection.

The most recent treatment method for herpes focuses on treating and preventing the illness with powerful medication.

1. Reduce the risk of instances of outbreaks

2. Reduce the pain caused by flares

3. Stop the spread of the disease to a person

The latest medications available to those suffering from Genital Herpes are

1. Valtrex

2. Famvir

3. Acyclovir

4. Dynamiclear

They are readily available in all nearby pharmacy retail stores and also at doctors. The final medication is among the most recent methods of treatment. It's the use of a topical treatment to treat those who are infected. This is due its popularity to the medication has anti-viral components like Sulphate, Hypericum, Aloe Vera, St. John's Wort and Vitamin E. Lysine is another supplement that is a source of amino acids which prevents the emergence of HSV in order to keep it in dormancy.

Natural Remedies to Cure Herpes

Although the current therapy of Genital Herpes proposes the suppression of the virus instead of any cure, the age-old natural remedies are backed by a myriad of evidences to support the effectiveness of permanent cure through it and the same.

1. Aloe Vera Gel/ Cream

If you are suffering from Genital Herpes with bursting clusters of lesions, the gel of aloe vera can be the most effective method to stop the outbreak. When applying the gel ensure that the affected area is dry. The best option is to choose to stay clear of bio-energetic herpes nodes that have homeopathic characteristics of the aloe Vera gel or cream.

2. Tea-Tree Oil/Cream

The antiseptic qualities of Tea-tree oil are known as is its powerful anti-viral properties. The oil must be sprayed to the affected area with the minimum of two times daily. Tea tree oil can help the lesions or blusters dry and heal quicker. This is among the most soothing options during the most severe cases of genital herpes.

3. Silica Gel

When silica gel that has been frozen is applied to an affected region, burning and itching stops. The organic silica gels when applied with adequate refrigeration, is among the top solutions for genital herpes.

4. St. John's Wort

The only natural ingredients that helps to stabilize depression and ease the sores that result from Genital Herpes, St. John's Wort is a long-standing natural remedy used in widespread usage.

5. Black Tea Bags and Lemon Bags

Applying cold tea bags, such as lemon bags can help reduce the burning, itching, and tingling that occur with Genital Herpes as well as its periodic recurrences. Sores and lesions are easily relieved when bathing or bathing in cold water or applying tea bags, but without cooling.

6. Intake of more vitamin C, Vitamin E and Zinc

To strengthen our immune system combat this herpes-related virus it is essential to take in plenty of Vitamin C, E, and Zinc within our daily diet. In the course of herpes the immune system is under an immediate threat, and it is essential to take care to ensure the immunity healthy.

7. Restricting sugar intake

Sugar is among the major immune system depressing elements , and therefore should be used within a certain limit.

8. Consuming Echinacea

Echinacea is among the oldest remedies to treat cold sores as well as Genital Herpes. It can be used to drink the juice, or used as an tincture.

9. Ayurveda

There are numerous ayurveda remedies that can be used to ease pain and to lessen the frequency and intensity of flares. The herbs that are used for the treatment are

1. Chandana

2. Devaduru

3. Ficus Plants

4. Utpala

5. Yesthimadu

6. Nagarmotha

7. Guduchi

8. Sariva

The above ingredients is to be mixed into the consistency of a powder. Take one teaspoon of the mixture to

* Boil over a moderate flame, along with 16 ounces water

* Boil until you have 4 ounces of liquid from the whole mixture

Apply it to the area affected and then rinse it off.

Or

Mix the powder with water, milk, and rose water.

Use this mixture to the infected areas.

Apply directly on infected areas after moistening it slightly.

1. Baking soda

One of the most effective dry-agents that can be used as a natural cure for Genital Herpes is baking soda. Baking soda aids in the evaporation of water from the affected lesions, allowing them to absorb and cleanse the sores properly.

2. Warm Bath

This is among the most effective ways to reduce the sensation of itching burning, and tingling within the affected region. Epson Salts and Domeboro are two essential elements to add to your bath. Each time, scrub the sores using soap to wash the blisters. If the affected region isn't fully soaked in warmer water it should be dried immediately. A hair dryer can aid those suffering from painful sores on their body to dry the infected areas.

3. Drinking Prunella Vulgaris as well as Rozites Caperata Mushrooms

Prunella Vulgaris is among the essential herbs that cure Genital herpes. It is used to treat the condition by utilizing its healing properties via warm bathing water to treat the sores that are cold. In addition, Rozites Caperata

Another type of mushroom that can be consumed to treat Genital Herpes.

4. Propolis Ointment

One of the primary factors in preventing and healing the spread from Genital Herpes blisters is the presence of propolis in the ointment form. The ideal concentration of propolis in the concoction must be 3percent. When applied to lesions, or to the area that is infected and in the surrounding area, heals lesions and blisters. The ointment is to be applied four times per day on the lesions , for at least 10 days.

5. Olive Oil

Use a teaspoon of Olive Oil and cook it in a pot , adding bee wax and lavender. Let the mixture cool and then apply it to the affected area. This is among the best natural cures to prevent the spread from Genital Herpes within measures.

6. The use of honey to treat Genital Herpes

One of the most effective medications to remittance to treat Genital Herpes, Honey should be used in excess similar to a bath with honey to cure Genital Herpes. Utilize raw, fresh honey to treat the condition and not the processed variety that can actually increase the disease further! Make sure to apply the honey on the affected lesions at least four times per day until lesions heal and crust. This is the most effective way to reduce and treat the genital and labial herpes.

7. Beware of Alcohol and Smoking

Another trigger that weakens immunity is the presence of alcohol, as well as nicotine. Avoid contact with nicotine and alcohol.

8. Utilizing Lubricants

When sexually intimate there is friction that results from dryness in the genital region can result in friction and Lubricants such as KY Jelly can aid in reducing the chance of cracking on the skin in the location. If it is cracked, it is also a sign of herpes that causes painful urination for a one or two weeks.

9. Intake of more fruits and minerals food items

Consumption of more minerals-rich foods and watery items helps to prevent dehydration of the body and boosts it to its maximum capacity. Bananas, strawberries and watermelon are among the top alternatives to fight Genital Herpes.

10. Food that is boring Bland Food

Another fantastic method to reduce dehydration within your body is to consume foods that are digested more quickly by your stomach . The presence of stomach cramps is not the only painful sign of the same.

11. Sufficient Salt

An effective way to keep your dehydration counter-techniques under control is by providing your body with enough salt within your regular diet. Salt pretzels and biscuits can be an excellent way to increase the amount of sweating you do. When the skin starts to chap and flake off because of dryness, applying a small amount of salt onto the face will help absorb the dryness away from the area, resulting with smoother and more supple skin. If you have itchy areas take a bath in salt water for a few minutes to alleviate itching and burning sensations that are felt in the lesions.

Chapter 11: Herpes The Lifelong Virus

Herpes often referred to also as Herpes Simplex, is a sexually transmitted virus. It's also a long-lasting disease, which means that it's an ongoing, permanent disease. A herpes-infected area appears to be a blister filled with pus. The physical signs are known as sores, but they look more like blisters.

SIGNS and SYMPTOMS HERPES

If you contract the herpes virus will be prone to outbreaks within a few days of being exposed sexually. Many people do not have symptoms, but have the disease, which makes them infectious. Patients who show frequent symptoms might experience symptoms often at first, but not so often in the future. Even though the symptoms decrease and do not become so severe, this is not a guarantee that the individual is free of herpes. In real life, he/she remains infectious and may spread the disease to anyone who comes in contact with or contact with bodily fluids. People who have been affected by the genital herpes virus are more likely to exhibit symptoms than those who have oral herpes.

The two types of HSV

There are two kinds of Herpes: HSV Type 1 and HSV Type 2. HSV1 is commonly called Oral Herpes; it is the more prevalent form that is afflicted by the condition. However HSV2 is known as Genital Herpes. There are various kinds of disorders or forms that are caused by Herpes Simplex viruses.

HSV-1 Oral Herpes

HSV Type 1 causes its disease predominantly around the mouth, however, it may extend to the face as well as the throat. In extreme instances, it may affect the area around your eyes.

HSV-2 Genital Herpes

HSV Type 2 infects the Genital region only. Both kinds of herpes can be be spread throughout the body.

Herpes is a highly infectious disease that is easily transferred through contact or saliva. It is transmitted through contact, particularly in the case or all of the body fluids of an affected or infected individual. Today there isn't a permanent treatment for herpes. once someone is infected, it'll be in their body for the rest of all of his or her life. The signs aren't always forever, but they can cause recurrent skin infections that can cause breakouts. They tend to be more frequent in cases where the defense system has been compromised.

THE IMPACTS OF HERPES

In addition to the embarrassment, anxiety and guilt that result from Herpes transmission people also suffer physical discomfort. People who contract the genital herpes virus by sexual activity are likely to be prone to breakouts. Typically, the signs will appear between 4 and 7 days following the infection. They appear as ulcers, blisters or blisters. In the case of genital herpes, they can be followed by the following symptoms:

* Vaginal discharge

* Pain when you urinate

* A feverish or feverish sensation

* Malaise

* Cold sores that are located around the mouth

* Blisters that are red

Red blisters are by far the most painful aspect of the flare. There may feel burning or tingling around the genital areas prior to the appearance of blisters. If they do, they'll expand across the entire genital area, from the outside to the buttocks, thigh as well as the rectum. They'll pop up over time and then will leave the person with the wounds. The symptoms won't last longer than 10 days, at the most and the ulcers can result in cuts. They will heal over time and will not leave a lot of scars.

What Herpes is affecting the Infected Person

Because the signs and symptoms of herpes are evidently unattractive and unpleasant to observe It is normal for those who are infected to feel depressed by the disease.

Low SELL-ESTEEM

Herpes sufferers is not only afflicted with the pain when they scream, and even if one does not suffer from it, that person is likely to be viewed as unpopular because of it. Since herpes can be transmitted and spreads through the body, a person with it is likely to have trouble finding a partner that is willing to accept the fact that they have them or. Although there are feelings of affection or love an individual with herpes will almost never be able to avoid due to the anxiety about transmission.

ARGENT or SELF-HATRED

If someone inherits herpes from someone else, specifically from a partner in love is likely to feel shame, even if they do not feel a sense of resentment for their partner. It's normal to experience this since herpes is a chronic disease that is yet to have any cure. While relationships might be running smoothly, there's no guarantee that they'll endure long or be capable of embracing that the illness exists on either side. A very difficult situations that can happen to those suffering from herpes is when they are left by their partner because of it. Some leave due to the suspicion being cheated on by their spouses while some are simply because of fear or displeasure. In this case the problem is not just a cause of depressing feelings and low self-esteem but also an outlet for self-hatred and anger at the person.

GUILT

Certain people may not resort to self-hatred, as some do, or blame their partner or someone else for acquiring herpes. Most of the time, the reason for sadness, depression and regret as well as other negative emotions is guilt. This guilt is caused from the thought of wanting to have learned better. The feeling of guilt is extremely unpleasant and is able to take root in the mind and linger for a long time. negativity, which can prevent the growth of happiness completely.

Acceptance and Coping

The results are a string or a string of events. There is first the breaking up of a relationship , or the trust, love or spark that a relationship has. After that, there is a sense of loneliness when telling the truth as well as keeping the secrets. The person is feeling different and less valuable or the impression that they are less valuable when compared to the other family or friends. The result is a decrease in interaction with new acquaintances and friends. In the end, you will experience a decrease in appetite or the lack of interest in everyday things like hobbies, enthusiasm for work, or aspirations.

START Taking IT CAREFULLY

Start one step at a. The first thing you realize is that there's no point in blameing you as well the individual who has infected you with herpes. The action has taken place and the effects have been manifested. The condition is not permanent, but it is possible to be a part of it. Many sufferers already have and continue to live and doing perfectly with HSV. It may be difficult initially however it will become better as time passes, so long as you are able to avoid outbreaks and control the symptoms.

LOVE, FORGIVE, and BE Kind to Yourself

Be kind to yourself. it will lead to positive thinking and the ability to find ways to live a happy life despite having herpes. Accept whatever error or mishap caused the illness. Herpes is an important factor in a person's life that should not be overlooked however it shouldn't determine the person as an individual or the life of others. Don't criticize, degrade or devalue yourself in order that others won't be able to do the same. If you can, invest your the effort into establishing self-esteem, regardless of how hard or difficult it might seem. This will be the foundation for becoming truly content.

SELF-RESPECT

When self-respect is established increase self-esteem by seeking support and comfort from others who can know the circumstances. People with STDs are unable to receive the moral support they need from loved ones and consequently, they get depressed over it. What they are missing is the help and encouragement from the people who are their most important loved ones - family. They are the ones who are likely to be able to understand and accept instantly any person suffering from herpes. The support of genuine friends can aid in emotional healing. However, be certain to select wisely whom you can help you and not create more stress for you.

Forgive and let go

When forgiveness acceptance, acceptance, self-esteem and self-esteem are built It is now possible to go on and enjoy life in the same way as the way it was before. The people who suffer from STDs are encouraged to continue doing the things that they love be focused on the things that make them happy and also pursue their careers. Herpes is a problem that affects people in a very limited way however it shouldn't be a factor into the way of living in general. You shouldn't quit dating anyone due to it. Take herpes as a normal part of your life that requires attention and maintenance. It is not embarrassing or something to be embarrassed about. It's only a rare disease that you do not intend to pass to anyone else but it's not the foundation of your character or your life. Take your own path and live your life to the highest degree.

Getting Through the Day With the Help of Others

While the signs or symptoms last for a long time however, they're not forever and are manageable. Though the emotional and mental effects of herpes are difficult to recover from however, there is an option to live a harmonious life in spite of the fact that it exists. There are many ways to be able to one to get over the negative consequences of the herpes virus. In reality, you can even accept herpes without feeling guilty about your self.

GET DIAGNOSED

The first thing to remember is that it isn't advisable to draw conclusions about the possibility of having herpes just by concluding that you have it based on symptoms you find on the web. Always consult with a professional medical professionals. Make an appointment for a consultation or visit an obstetrician to have any suspected blisters examined. If the test results come back positive for HSV Don't be depressed consult your doctor or the OB-GYN on how to deal with the outbreaks. If you have questions you have in your head Do not be afraid to talk to your doctor and gather the most information you can. The more you understand about HSV the easier and more effective to manage the situation and accept it.

SUBSCRIBE TO A SUPPORT GROUP

You're not alone Accept and recognize the fact. There are many who have been affected by herpes, both in a way, either unknowingly or with a conscious effort. Although the condition can cut you off from people who surround you to a certain extent, it is not a reason to shouldn't be a reason to cut off your access to the world. There are others who comprehend what you're experiencing and feeling at the moment. Many are going through the exact similar issues, while others have overcome it, and they have advice on how to overcome. There are groups that cater to those with sexually transmitted illnesses such as herpes. Look up these groups and then join one to find out more about managing the disease.

There is no end to the possibilities in seeking help or support. The presence of your loved ones will be enough evidence that you're not all alone. While your partner might choose to leave the relationship, family members members and acquaintances will not be as harsh or cold toward you. In reality there are a lot of people who are willing to accept those suffering from sexually transmitted disorders. They're not widespread, however, they're not uncommon also. If there's nobody physically and emotionally supportive, there's every option for seeking counselling and compassion via STD help groups. They seek acceptance, acceptance and acceptance, as well as the elimination of self-doubt and guilt, and the reinvigoration confidence in self and love for self.

SEEK A THERAPIST

If joining the support group isn't doing the trick or is difficult, you have the option of consulting the help of a therapy session. For some , it might appear unimportant however the truth is that it's far from unnecessary or ineffective. Herpes' symptoms can ravage the mental and emotional well-being. When depression is at its peak individuals with STDs do not only feel sad but they also become more vulnerable to mental illnesses as a portion sufferers fall into physical and social solitude. Some even experience suicidal thoughts due to how people feel about their bodies as well as their bodies.

Support Groups in contrast to. Therapists

Support groups can aid in easing those feelings of self-hatred with the assistance of similar individuals. If there is no one to connect with or speak to, an affected person is bound to stifle the emotions and thoughts until they become overwhelming and explode. A therapist, on contrary, though not a person with whom you can connect, they can offer suggestions and listen. A therapist will help you expose your thoughts and emotions until they are released to the root source of the problem.

True that therapists will evaluate the patient after just a few sessions, but this doesn't mean they'll prescribe drugs immediately. This is contingent upon the severity of the circumstance. There are instances where STD patients are so anxious or depressed that they become exasperated that medications will require. In addition the counselor can determine what you'll need the most. The therapist will guide you through what kind of activities can best distract you, or how to manage negative thoughts using positive thinking, and other methods.

Get Healthy Through Healthy Living

A healthy lifestyle isn't simply mean that you can exercise regularly. A healthy lifestyle requires an individual to be committed to a healthy lifestyle, especially for someone who is suffering from the effects of herpes it's vital to take the necessary steps.

Why LIVEING HEALTHY COUNTERS HERPES IS IMPORT

Many people believe that living a healthy life is a standard best for everyone that doesn't have any significant benefits to those who are specifically "disabled" such as those suffering from STDs. However, a healthy lifestyle can be more beneficial to people who are affected in one way or other. As mentioned before herpes outbreaks can occur in situations of low immunity or those who are constantly stressed. When you live a healthy lifestyle, stress-related outbreaks will not only diminish, but will almost disappear.

Dietary Health

A healthy lifestyle can provide a healthy body as well as an improved immune system that helps to reduce the frequency and herpes recurrence. There are studies of healthy eaters who have reported having an

80% lower risk of developing herpes than those who consume sugary and fatty foods. Simply simply, a balanced and balanced diet that is healthy and nutritious and regular exercise, paired with a positive mindset can ensure a healthy body and a more positive mind.

Exercising Regularly

You will be amazed by the effects of endorphins. Naturally, people affected by herpes or its symptoms are so depressed emotionally that they cease to be proactive completely. If they are proactive again or even only the second time you will be able to significantly lessen the stress that comes with transmitting herpes. It's not just good mentally for the person, it can also be beneficial in terms of physical.

Stress Reduction

Herpes outbreaks are common, but occur frequently and more severe in stressful times for those suffering from the disease and can be accompanied by lower immunity. By exercising and reducing stress, these breakouts can be significantly reduced and avoided when someone is sick. Therefore, do yourself a favor and engage in engaging in enjoyable physical exercises. While it may not be distracting and substitute for the lack of a connection, it'll also ensure a healthy health for your body and positive vibes for your mind.

How do you manage and reduce Outbreaks

On PRODUCTIVITY and SEX

It is possible to enjoy an active sexual life after having an STD such as herpes. There are methods to be able to enjoy or end your sex lifestyle without passing the disease on to anyone else. Some individuals may consider it necessary to keep their illness secret but not let loved ones inform them of their condition to avoid an eventuality. Some who prefer the approval of their partners prior to engaging in sexual sex. In any case, it's essential to wear protective products like condoms, in the event of sex with someone else.

This can stop spreading the illness and help keep your loved ones protected. For those suffering from oral herpes it's beneficial to use dental dams as well as other similar products so as to avoid being a source of infection. Consult with an OB-GYN doctor or physician about the products that can be used to protect against herpes from spreading to other people. If there is an outbreak of herpes at time, it is crucial to avoid any physical or sexual contact with anyone else since she is considered to be the highest infectious phase in the course of disease. To alleviate any anxiety that result from this lack of sleep opt to distract your self through exercise or hobbies. This will help you relax however it will also satisfy your sexual desires and give you a sense of accomplishment.

CUT DOWN ALCOHOL

As it is essential to lead a healthy life that is why there is no reason to hold off on the reduction of drinking alcohol. There are some instances when those with herpes develop flares after drinking alcohol or who drink regularly. Although this can be distinct for every person however, there is a good possibility that alcohol could trigger an outbreak, and may even prolong it. This can add to the stressors you have that you are facing right now that will make you feel more stressed. If you drink, do it slowly and with care.

Keep a food journal

Keep a record of your food choices. This may sound like a joke, but it can be very beneficial in the management of herpes outbreaks. The trigger for outbreaks as well as the severity and frequency is different for each individual. The most common cause is specific food items that can trigger reactions in an infected person. It's similar to an allergic reaction but can trigger Herpes-related outbreaks. Like we said earlier, the majority of people experience more outbreaks because of alcoholism. Some sufferers have herpes recurrence as a result of caffeine, while other people have outbreaks after eating nuts.

It is impossible to know the exact food that can trigger an unusual or sudden outbreak. The food journal can assist in identifying which foods to avoid in order to reduce the consequences of herpes. You can think of it as health maintenance to prevent illness. In the end, it's an illness that must be taken care of and monitored to ensure better health overall.

Adopt the habit of being clean and CLEAN

One of the toughest issues to overcome or accept is that the herpes virus makes you feel completely clean in a variety of ways. The cold sores and blisters are not pleasant to look at and even more uncomfortable to feel. If not washed or clean, they become more infectious and may spread to the skin's the surface. Patients suffering from herpes tend to be so depressed by their perform their duties that they neglect to take care of their bodies, and then unknowingly allow the blisters to appear throughout the body. While it may be painful for some people, shower one to twice a day, especially when the outbreak is only beginning. This can lessen the impact as well as the sweltering and itchy rashes. It will also stop it from spreading throughout the skin. Additionally, it can help to reduce the time between outbreaks.

GET PRESCRIPTION DRUGS

If you suspect or believe there is a possibility that an outbreak of herpes may be likely to occur or is already occurring, it's ok to ask for an appointment with your physician. There are certain kinds of medicines that can prevent the outbreak, reduce its duration, or alleviate the blisters or pain the outbreak causes. It is also beneficial to take an intake of vitamin supplements regularly at least every day. This helps to regulate the imbalances in hormones and chemicals in the body which could cause the outbreaks.

Chapter 12: The General Characteristics

And Features Of Germ Of Lip Herpes.

The lip herpes germs are part of the family known as herpes viruses. also known as herpes virus of the 1st type and the 2nd types (HSV-1 as well as HSV-2) also known as herpes simplex virus. In this case, the herpes virus in the 2nd type is the most likely to cause symptoms of herpes that occurs in the region of the genital organs and can cause the lips to swell only in rare instances. Contrarily the herpes virus of the type 1 causes lip blisters in over 90 percent of instances.

Herpes simplex viruses are part of the DNA-containing virus type. According to researchers the vision (the virus particle that contains the genetic information and is surrounded by the coat of proteins) is composed of 74 genes that code for 84 different proteins.

The virus infects the human body via mucous membranes' epithelium. In rare instances, it is transmitted via skin injuries. Once it has reached the nucleus and the genetically-controlled device of any cell the virus inserts its DNA-code within the DNA of the cell and causes it to produce DNA and proteins for the creation of new virus. In cells, fresh viruses form and are then dispersed through cells that are neighboring or by the blood stream throughout the body.

Axons of nerve cells are able to become infected and remain within the body for a long time. In general, this viral depots form in the spinal ganglions, which are areas with the highest concentration of large nerve cells.

After the virion is in the cell, as soon as two hours following the time that new proteins from outside appear in it the number of proteins is maximum around 8 hours following.

The herpes virus is replicated in any cell like this, but the cloning process of viral particles takes place the fastest in epithelial cells, which are cells from mucous membranes lymph , and blood.

The rapid growth of viral particles in blood can lead, as a consequence, to the external manifestations of the herpes. Over the course of several days our body's defense system carries to provide the proper reaction to the infection. Through the use of various defense mechanisms, the majority of viruses that are present in the body are eradicated and the remnants of the virus persist in the genetically adapted apparatus of nerve cells.

The latent stage starts with the virions that are produced by nerve cells are destroyed quickly through the system of immunity. only after the immune system weakens their reproduction may go out of hand and symptoms typical of the first infection could manifest over and over.

Lip herpes causes and methods for carrying on the infection

The main causes of the herpes are either the initial infection of the patient by the virus , or weakening the immune system, resulting in consequent relapse.

In rare instances there is no distinctive symptoms, even following the first infection. It is usually the case when a patient is infected by the herpesvirus of another type because of the overlap of various antibodies, the virus is "annihilated" through immune mechanisms.

The most common causes of relapses are of the time:

* Different diseases that are somatic which include chronic conditions ranging from diabetes to influenza

• Intoxication in the human body

* Stress

* Exhaustion, physical debilitation

* Alcohol addiction, addiction to drugs and smoking cigarettes

* Undernourishment

* Menstruation in women

In certain cases, signs of herpes may manifest for other reasons. For instance following overheating in the sun or when drinking strong coffee.

Herpes Simplex is a virus that can be often transmitted following intimate contact that occurs between the carriers and recipient, whether through kisses, sexual interactions, or simple gestures.

Furthermore, there are alternatives to carrying herpes:

* Airborne through the air, whether it's sneezing or talking

* With tangible objects like dishes, towels, and clothes.

* From the mother to the baby during childbirth

In this case, the most common and well-known method of passing on the disease is to share the interaction of adult patients in the stage of relapse with children (sometimes after the completion of this stage, there aren't any visible signs). The mother is usually the primary source of the infection. If a child is infected with herpes in the first few months of its life because of the immunity it received from its mother, in the later years, the number of immunoglobulins diminishes and the child is more prone to infection.

Nearly all people are susceptible to the virus. There are, however, a few instances that make up 3-4 percent of the population. People with inborn mechanisms for defending themselves from the virus. Scientists aren't sure the mechanism that works, but the reality is that they aren't affected by the herpes virus.

Risk groups: who often contract the lip herpes?

Relapses of herpes that is followed by all the unpleasant signs associated with the love blister typically occurs to those who suffer from:

* The susceptibility to allergies.

* Immune deficiencies, including HIV-positive

*The immune system is was suppressed in response to therapeutic methods

* Infectious illnesses

* The propensity to drink and smoking cigarettes.

The first disease and, as a result, the acute illness usually occur between 3 and 4 years old when the child begins engaging with a lot of people. This means that he/she will have greater chances of coming across those who carry herpes.

Signs and symptoms of the lips herpes

The lip herpes is a condition that has many distinct symptoms, which must be listed in the order that they manifest in the course of the disease. The entire course of treatment from their first appearance until their complete disappearance of the disease can be divided into various phases:

1. Itching and mild reddening. After the initial infection itching can occur between 7 and 30 weeks after infection is introduced in the human body. In this stage it is possible to not feel any symptoms but they'll be an accurate indicator of the infection. Along with a slight tingling sensation on the lips, there is the possibility of having itching all over your face. The duration of this condition can range from a few hours up to a couple of days and during this time you can avoid the progression of the disease through the help of medicines.

2. The prodromal stage. The areas in which you felt tingling begin swelling , and tiny transparent bubbles begin to appear on the surface. After a while, the bubbles begin to expand and then become cloudy. Pressure builds up in them and they can become extremely painful.

3. Within a few days, the bubbles begin to explode and then are replaced by blisters, which are soon overshadowed in a scab. The blistering process is quite common over a period of one day. dry scabs only appear as

a substitute for bubbles. In this time, the patient is the most contagious.

4. The time of full recovery of blisters. It can last up to up to 4-5 days. In rare cases, small marks following the largest blisters may be left on the lips. At this point, you may occasionally feel pain and itching in the healing areas.

5. Regeneration of the skin to replace blisters that were previously present. It can last for about a week. In rare instances, the relapse may recur at this point.

It is not common, however there are symptoms like fever, sickness or general fatigue. In general they are temporary and fade on the stage of the bubbles.

The possibility of complications after the herpes lip

The most common complications that occur after herpes are that are caused by the herpes virus itself , but only in areas that are not previously affected by it. For instance, if the patient rubs their eyes during the acute phase, the virus may infiltrate the mucous membranes of the eye. Upon the active reproduction , it could cause ophthalmic herpes that may result in the loss of vision, or total blindness.

The virus is often found onto lips and hands due to which herpetic eczema is seen. Sexual contact with the mouth during the relapse could result in the transmission of herpes that affect the sexual organs as well as the development of herpes genital.

The medical profession has been able to identify a variety of conditions for which lip herpes was the most prominent ethological cause:

* Encephalitis, meningitis

* Gingivitis, stomatitis , and other conditions that affect the oral cavity

* Disorders of the ear throat and nose Tonsillitis, laryngitis vestibular disorders, pharyngitis the otitis process and hearing disorders

* Prostatitis, Urethritis and the inability of spermatozoids to males

* Endometritisand amnionitis metroendometritis. coleitis and infertility among women.

* Iridocyclitis and keratitis. It can also cause optic neuritis, phlebempraxis the chorioretinitis

* Pneumonia

* Myocarditis and myocarditis

* HSV-lymphoadenopathy

* Hepatitis, colitis proctitis

• Depression and aggravation in schizophrenic patients

In many instances, these problems aren't connected to the herpes lip because people aren't paying at all. In the same way it is important to make the right and timely diagnosis of herpes could help to protect your body from serious issues.

Diagnostics for the herpes on the lips

In most cases herpes is diagnosed based on visual signs following a thorough examination and interviewing on the part of the sufferer. In the initial stage of the disease or after a relapse, there is a chance to be mistakenly identifying the herpes as any of the following conditions:

* Impetigo is caused by bacteria, and characterized by herpetic bubbles shaped like blisters may appear on lips

* Atopic dermatitis that is most commonly on the lips

* Sprue that causes blisters in the mouth

In instances, where doctors are afraid of making a mistake in the diagnostics using visuals or it is necessary to test for the existence of the virus within the body during the stage of latent, they utilize more accurate and precise techniques:

1. IFA - immune ferment analysis. It's used to detect antigens IgM as well as IgG for the herpesvirus in blood. If they're found this indicates It is likely that your body had contact with the herpesvirus (except in cases involving infants younger than 6 months). This method does not allow for the differentiation of the herpes virus of 1st type from that of the virus of the 2nd type.

2. PCR - polymerase chain reaction. It's used to find DNA from the herpes virus in the sample used for analysis, including blood, mucous membranes, spit or amniotic fluids.

3. Immunofluorescence reaction.

Usually blood from the patient is utilized for all of these tests. The blood sample is taken from an empty stomach, and it is recommended to avoid eating a lot of heavy meals prior to the test.

Cure for herpes on the lips using pharmaceuticals

Treatment of herpes of the lips generally is a result of weakening the virus in the initial phase of the disease and then a relapse with the intention of preventing the development of complications, as well as stopping the symptoms that are distinct from each other. It is difficult to remove herpes virus. In theory, even the total regeneration of blood in the body will not be effective since the DNA of the virus is stored in the nervous cells, which will continue to be created by herpes virus virions.

The most popular anti-herpes medication currently is Aciclovir/Zovirax. It is the alternative to desoxigunozyne which is the main DNA component. The scientist who developed this drug received the Nobel Prize for its development and in the present, several highly-popular medications are manufactured using Aciclovir. There are:

* Zovirax is one of the most well-known gels to treat herpes around the globe

* Aciclovir Acri

* Aciclovir AST

* Valaciclovir

Another well-known pharmaceutical used for treating herpes is Famciclovir. Famvir.

Zovirax and Panavir Gel are extremely effective if you apply them to the area of irritation at the beginning of the acute herpes prior to when the first bubbles appear on your lips. If you apply the gel on your lips frequently, the disease will not develop. But, at the point where bubbles begin to appear they will not be as effective but they can accelerate the healing of blisters.

Valaciclovir is the strongest medication than the others, but unlike Famvir, it's not available without a prescription from a doctor. As with Zovirax in pill form are used when the illness is serious. Valaciclovir can be taken two times: when the first signs of symptoms, in the form of 4 pills. The second dose is taken 12 hours following the initial dose. If you take the medication within the first 12 hours after the moment of relapse the primary symptoms of the disease will not appear.

There are now vaccinations available to lower the risk of relapses from lip herpes, however the scientific research hasn't confirmed their efficacy.

To alleviate pain in the herpes virus, you can make use of painkillers that are weak like lidocaine, articaine and benzocaine.

In alternative medicine they usually use sea buckthorn oil or pet rose oil aloe juice, or the Kalanchoe juice, as well as an zinc potion. The potions are applied on the outer edge of the affected area and afterward - inside, so as not to cause smears from the bubbles onto healthy skin.

The herpes on the lips can occur during pregnancy as well as breastfeeding

Particular attention must be given to the issue of lip herpes during nursing and pregnancy.

The symptoms of lip herpes do not cause abortion, nor are they the reason that makes women stop breastfeeding. In addition, the herpes virus isn't passed down from mother to child and is not a factor in the fertility of a man by itself. However, the appearance the love blisters on the woman who is pregnant is the ultimate indicator of an immune system that is weak and is a signal to identify the causes for this shrinking. In some instances, especially severe herpes may cause miscarriage.

If the mother experiences symptoms of herpes during her breastfeeding period, she must follow these guidelines for baby treatment:

* Wash your hands prior to touching the baby

* Put on the dressing in bulk for feeding and swaddling the baby

* Avoid kisses as they are among one of the main causes transmitting the herpes virus.

In the treatment of herpes on the mother's pregnancy, anti-herpes medications for the childbirth period should not be taken. Zovirax and other medications are available only as gels to be used externally and their constituents are not in the bloodstream and do not affect the growth of the fetus nor in the composition of milk.

The prevention of Lip herpes

To reduce the chance of contracting herpes infection , or to lower the chances of relapses, you should adopt specific measures for prevention of the herpes lip infection:

* Avoid contact with persons who have obvious signs of the herpes virus.

It is not recommended to share personal items, like your toothbrush, dish towels or clothes with anyone else.

* To prevent inappropriate sexual encounters, and in particular oral kisses

* To ensure that you do not overheat in the sun or cooling too much however, simultaneously, constantly temper yourself to boost the power of your body to protect itself from external shocks.

* To promptly and effectively manage emerging somatic illnesses

* To maintain an active lifestyle, take healthy meals, keep yourself in check and exercise regularly

The special vaccinations are not part of the prevention of lip herpes. Herpetic vaccines that are polyvalent have proven their ineffectiveness in the context of specific experiments and vaccinations against Genital Herpes aren't particularly efficient against the herpes of the lips and are completely useless for males. The reason is that the medicine hasn't developed a method to help you fight herpes completely.

Similar measures must be used to prevent herpes among children. The child should be separated from any family members with evident signs of lip herpes. He or should be given nutritious food, and any new health issues must be treated immediately. If you are able to count on that if your child develops the herpes virus, it will trigger the first onset of the virus swiftly and without any consequences.

The Body Herpes and its various forms features and methods of Cure

The term "body herpes" is an ambiguous word. The illness that is called "herpes" is typically visible on the lips or the genital area as well as causing flares in other parts of the body, but only in rare instances. Other viruses tend to be more aggressive in this respect and cause massive effects on the skin, and obvious blisters.

In the vast majority of instances, the causes for the herpetic eruptions that occur on the body stem from the decline of the patient's immunity as well as the recurrence of the disease that he or she had to overcome in the past, possibly quite a long time back.

However, the initial infection by herpetic virus causes the appearance of the typical eruptions and blisters. The kind of herpes has an impact on the nature, size and the severity of flares that appear on your body.

Herpetic viruses of various types that produce skin eruptions

There are over 200 of these herpetic viruses there are six viruses that are the most prevalent among human beings and can cause a rash to the body. They comprise:

1. Herpes simplex virus is of the first kind. The majority of the time, this is what results in lip eruptions which are known in the form of "love bumps". If it's transferred to other body parts it may cause irritations and inflammations around the area of the eyes (on the eyelids and eyebrows) behind the nails or in the groin within the mouth, and in very rare cases in the skins of the other body areas.

2. The Herpes Simplex virus is of the 2nd kind which is extremely similar to the one previously mentioned, however it is found in the majority of cases in the groin . It

causes eruptions on the sexual organs, in the area in the stomach, on the buttocks and hips, but not always on the legs and back.

3. The chicken pox virus causes known chicken pox the time of initial infection, accompanied by a massive swelling, distinctive rash that covers the entire body. In the event of a relapse, it can lead to shingles that are characterized by skin abrasions on the sides of the torso, or in the lower back.

4. Epstein-Barr virus causing infectious mononucleosis. In its normal type, this illness doesn't cause skin rashes but the use of antibiotics in the treatment of diseases that are developing in conjunction with it usually results in a rash on the body.

5. Cytomegalovirus It is extremely common within humans. Skin blisters can occur in very rare instances and only if the immune system is weak.

6. Herpes virus is of 6th kind that can cause the pseudo-rubella. The most prominent manifestation of this disease is the massive

skin rash that covers the entire body, mostly in infants and children, that looks like that of rubella.

The body's eruptions are typical for the threat of exotic monkey herpes, which is not often transmitted to humans. However, in the event of infection, it usually can cause death.

Herpes simplex virus and the specifics of body itchy rash

The body herpes caused by herpes simplex virus comes with numerous distinctive characteristics that allow to detect it quickly.

The rash that is caused by the herpes simplex virus resembles an abundance of tiny liquid bubbles, which are initially transparent before changing to a light whitish color in the course of the illness.

The method of infection and the location where the virus first reaches the virus within the body, the eruptions could be seen in different areas of the body.

* On lips.

* On the genitalia, inside the groin, and sometimes in the vagina of women, or on the surface of the rectum, both women and men.

* On buttocks, frequently after contracting sexually transmitted herpes in anal sex.

* In the region of the eyes, including the conjunctiva. This causes herpetic conjunctivitis.

• Behind the nails, or within the area of the cuticle. In this situation, the disease is known as herpetic-whitlow.

• On your neck, or ear for athletes who engage in contact sports. This condition is known as "fighters herpes" and, in addition to eruptions, can be characterized by the symptoms of fever.

* The hair growth line is located near the scalp and causing the flow of dandruff as well as the continuous itching of the skin on the head.

* On the skin folds, such as knees, elbows, in the abdomen, which can cause scratches-like wounds. This kind of appearance is

common among those with a weak immune system or serious immune deficiency.

* As eczema-like bumps everywhere on the body of those suffering from dermatitis.

It should be noted that besides the these three instances, all other cases are very uncommon. The eruptions of the genitalia and lips can be a real problem for those affected by the herpes syphilis virus. They often are seen during the colder season of the year. They cause not only an less attractive appearance, but also some severe, and sometimes fatal, complications.

Chicken pox as well as the shingles

The virus that causes chicken pox (varicella zoster) is most prevalent in children younger than eight years old and causes the well-known chicken pox. Like other herpes virus are, it is not completely eliminated in the body, and once it has infected, it is left in the nervous tissue. Due to the weakening of immunity this virus can trigger shingles at any time.

The chicken pox eruptions in the body are easily diagnosed and cause great pain for the sufferer. They're usually painful and itchy. When scratched out they develop into tiny blisters and cuts that are more painful, and they become gateways to different infections.

Additionally, although eruptions don't leave any trace after the disease, if they're scratched and scabs appear as visible marks after recovery.

The chicken pox outbreaks can be seen across the body. They appear like normal pink spots. The part of them turns into pimples that contain the transparent liquid. They typically occur between two and three weeks after infection.

When the initial flare, the rash is gone completely but the subsequent diminution in the immunity system implies that it could reappear in a different form and another set of symptoms known as herpes zoster or shingles. The most prominent features of it are:

* The tiny area that is affected. It is often an area with a pink-colored scratch in the face. Its size is comparable to an average palm.

* A unilateral ailment on the body. The rash can be seen on the left and on the left or on the other side of the shoulders, back the neck, and is more common on the legs and arms.

The absence of blisters. The rash appears as if it has scratch marks on your skin.

The risk of shingles is that when it's severe, it can lead to serious complications, and in many instances it can cause post-herpetic neurogia very painful at the sites of eruptions that have not completely gone after months, weeks and even years.

Roseola Infantum: signs and risk.

This condition is most commonly seen in infants and is marked by large eruptions on the body that resemble flares that occur during rubella. It's preceded by signs of fever. Its complications could be caused by crunches on the baby , or the an outbreak of meningitis or encephalitis.

The roseola rash itself can trigger flares that are caused by the virus known as herpes simplex however they are more focused and bright red. They don't cause as much itching as the rash that occurs during chicken pox but they can make babies suffer in the same way. They will disappear on their own, without any further treatment within 4-7 days.

The nature of the rash in the course of an infection caused by Epstein-Barr virus and the cytomegalovirus

The eruptions of the skin are not common symptoms of the two viruses. In general, cytomegalovirus does not show any apparent symptoms on patients. Also when the immune system is weak, it can cause the symptoms of mononucleosis which are remarkably like the infection mononucleosis that occurs after contracting the Epstein-Barr virus.

Excessive skin eruptions in these diseases often occur when a patient is prescribed antibiotics. It is important to know that antibiotics aren't effective in curing these diseases since all of antibiotics do nothing in combating viruses. In some rare cases that have mononucleosis or the mononucleosis-syndrome may manifest with various other illnesses that are treatable with antibiotics.

In these instances the rash may not be obvious; it typically is seen on the sides, hips and around the Genital organs. It's not painful, and will usually go away within just a few days.

Different types of herpes are diagnosed in accordance with body eruptions

Based on the body's eruptions, period and the accompanying signs of virus, herpes viral diseases are distinct from one another, and in a few cases do they leave doubt and the possibility of a error to be made.

Therefore, if the eruptions occur on tiny areas of the body, such as the lips' surfaces and eyelids, or on the cuticles on nails - then one could be talking about herpes simplex. The visible signs of herpes simplex are the transparency or the clouds of bubbles.

The same clear or cloudy bubbles, however, that have appeared on the genitalia, hips or groin, indicate the existence of the herpes simplex virus with its genital variant.

If the eruptions of the same color appear throughout the body and aren't located in the area of the genitalia, but are associated with lymphatic vessels swelling, it's possible to identify mononucleosis as well as cytomegalovirus. It can be difficult to distinguish these two conditions and, for this reason you should employ specific tests for diagnosing a disease in the lab.

The red eruptions are usually a sign of roseola infantum or chicken pox. In the case of the first the dissociation of blisters is typical. Chicken pox can affect all children. The second illness is more prone to infants and infants under 2 years old. Additionally, the roseola rash is characterised by large body areas that are completely covered in itchy rash.

The most accurate diagnosis can be made using special laboratory methods. In any event, making the diagnosis to determine the next treatment must be carried out only by a qualified doctor, as attempts to diagnose yourself often result in a mistake and, consequently is the result of ineffective and sometimes dangerous self-treatment.

Why is body herpes so dangerous?

In addition to the body eruptions that occur, most herpes virus are distinguished by the possibility to cause serious complications. There are a few of them:

Prostatitis, herpetic cystitis cracks of the rectum herpetic urethritis that occurs in the genital herpes

* Myocarditis and encephalitis the pyoderma syndrome, the time of chickenpox or shingles.

* Affections and inflammations of internal organs due to cytomegaloviral infection in patients with immune deficiency

* Growth of tumors that are cancerous because of the infection of the Epstein-Barr virus.

Meningitis and Encephalitis at children in the roseola

However, complications from herpes arc the most serious when herpetic rash develops on the time of conception. Based on the type of disease or the time in which eruptions are visible and the nature of the disease the fetus could be affected by virus and may also experience some variations in its development, all the way up to miscarriage and death.

In truth, it occurs very rarely, however this possibility makes doctors keep track of all herpetic virus infections at pregnant women and make necessary precautions at the appropriate the right time.

Treatment of body herpes: drugs and techniques

Cure for the body herpes relies on the virus itself that can cause eruptions. Utilization of specific, robust pharmaceuticals is recommended only when due to the emergence of the infection , severe complications could be a possibility. In general, it is seen in pregnant women, individuals with immune deficiencies , as well as at newborn infections.

Herpes or herpes virus the 3rd type appears suddenly in the body, and the effectiveness of treatment is directly dependent on how quickly the treatment has started. If you notice the first signs of herpes eruptions, you must take the following steps:

Anti-viral anti-herpetic drugs like Acyclovir, Zovirax, Valtrex, Virolex. They are typically manufactured as pills to be consumed orally however, in certain cases doctors may prescribe injections of such drugs. It is essential to take anti-viral medicines prior to the there are bubbles appearing, at the level of the increased skin sensitiveness.

Antiviral medications for external use, like gels, creams and sprays like Herperax, Acyclovir, Zovirax and Viru-Mertz Serol. These medications should be applied to the affected areas each 3-4 times per day. Before sleep, it's best to wash the anti-herpes cream , and then change it onto the antiseptic.

Painkillers and non-steroid anti-inflammatory medications such as ibuprofen and paracetamol. Creams that contain lidocain or Acetaminofen are suggested for external use. It's hard to cure herpes with painkillers since the virus spreads through your peripheral nerve system.

Other methods. These include lotions (Depantenol, Pantenol spray) which help to strengthen the skin's cells and can help heal blisters.

Antiseptic medications. To avoid spreading of infection, it's advised to take antibiotics externally. Herpetic eruptions can be treated through Miramistin Chlorhexodin or streptocyde, or the zinc potion.

Local warming-up medications. To speed up the metabolism of tissues and, in certain instances warming-up medications such as those from the Vietnamese balm "Golden Star" or the cream for children "Doctor MOM" are employed. They also have anti-inflammatory and antiseptic effects.

Conclusion

A lot of people experience an overwhelming surge of emotions after being diagnosed. In the beginning, they might experience surprise or disbelief, accompanied by guilt and sorrow. As time passes, many are able to transition into acceptance, but they could be snubbed with the persistent suspicion that it's either way or another their fault and there is no permanent solution available to them. The fortunate ones can regain confidence in themselves and have the comfort of knowing that the herpes diagnosis does not mean that they have to alter their lives. However, there's more there! Herpes simplex is a common disease, as you are aware of. While it's not uncommon but the general scientific community insists that there isn't a cure for this condition. But, if you do a research for yourself , and take care of yourself by following the advice from this manual, you'll demonstrate your case and find that there's plenty of evidence that suggests otherwise. Finding ways to deal with the diagnosis of herpes is a significant stage in the healing process however, it doesn't need to be the point at which your journey comes to an end. Through this book, you've acquired a wealth of knowledge about the virus that causes herpes, the effects it has on human bodies, and standard treatment methods. Also, you have discovered the truth of what your doctor has not yet told you about this illness. Many people suffering from herpes think that it's an illness that will last forever there is hope in the distance. Following the guidelines in this book, you will be able to get rid of the herpes virus and enjoy the relief of lasting relief.

www.ingramcontent.com/pod-product-compliance
Lightning Source LLC
Chambersburg PA
CBHW060329030426
42336CB00011B/1258